Complete Fitness Trainer Certification: Beginner To Advanced

Gaurav Sanjiv Kalangan

Published by Gaurav Sanjiv Kalangan, 2024.

Also by Gaurav Sanjiv Kalangan

Learn Options Strategies Options Basics & Greeks For Stock Trading By Technical Analysis

Bitcoin, Altcoins & ICOs Learn the Basics of Digital Coins from Zero

Time Management This Is How I Work 300 Percent Faster

How To Build And Implement A Winning Pricing Strategy

Networking For Introverts: Gracefully Exiting A Conversation

Accounting 101: Learn Cost Accounting From A To Z

Growth Marketing: Strategy & Execution Bootcamp For Startups

Develop The Mental Strength Of A Warrior For Success In Life

Time Management Mastery: Productivity & Goals

Complete Fitness Trainer Certification: Beginner To Advanced

Table of Contents

Copyright 1

About.. 2

Why Are You Fat 3

Fat Burn Mantra... 8

Easy Fat Killer Technique 15

Yo-Yo Effect.. 19

Easy Yoga Practice..................................... 22

List of Fat-Pumping Foods To Avoid.......... 29

Fat Burn Supplement & Detox Plan............ 37

How To Get Rid Of Love Handles................ 55

Everyone Wants Success 60

Set BIG Goals... 61

Make Real Decisions................................... 65

Consistency Is Key...................................... 69

How To Be Accountable 73

Nothing Is Impossible 77

Live In The Moment 81

Being Adventurous 85

Words Of Success...89

Life-Long Learning..93

No Such Thing As Failure 97

Recap 101

Healthy Eating Lifestyle 102

Powerful Benefits of Eating Healthy.............105

Alkaline Foods vs Acidic 108

Understanding The Food Pyramid.................112

Food Cholesterol 117

Recommended Foods For Exceptional Health 122

Cooking Simple Healthy Meals.......................127

Guidelines To Well-being..................................132

Healthy Binge-Free Lifestyle 138

Terrifying Food Facts 139

Signs Of Compulsive Overeating....................142

Why You Lack Control Around Food 145

The Dangers Of Overeating.............................149

The 10 Types Of Overeating 153

Great Strategies To Prevent Overeating.........158

Overcoming An Overeating Disorder 165

Final Ideas & Tips 171

Proven Steps And Strategies 172

The Vegan Journey - Health & Vitality 174

Debunking Vegan Myths 179

Vegan Athletes - Plenty Of Muscle 184

Fueling The Vegan Warrior 188

Vegan Warrior Workout Plan 193

Going Vegan 198

Thoughts & Tips 202

Body & Mind Health Masterclass: A Complete Guide to BodyDetox 205

Expectations & Days 1-3 207

Enemas 209

Days 4-8 211

Energy levels 213

Restarting the System 214

Parasite Home Test 216

Elimination 217

An Emotional & Physical Journey 218

Products required..219

Defecation 222

Changes..224

Preparation 225

Documenting process 226

First days 227

Preparation for enema...229

Enema Demonstration..231

Apple Bonus...234

After the enema 235

Some words of encouragement 236

Day 4..237

Days 5-7 238

Days 8-11 240

Days 12-14 242

Coffee enema and passive weight loss............................244

Recipes? 246

Stick to it...247

Conclusion 248

Copyright

Published by Gaurav Sanjiv Kalangan

Copyright © 2024 Gaurav Sanjiv Kalangan

All rights reserved.

Distributed by Gaurav Sanjiv Kalangan

Complete Fitness Trainer Certification: Beginner To Advanced

Design and composition by Gaurav Sanjiv Kalangan Cover design by Gaurav Sanjiv Kalangan For permission credits.

To offset the number of trees consumed in the printing of our books, Gaurav Sanjiv Kalangan donates a portion of the proceeds from each printing to the Arbor Day Foundation. Gaurav Sanjiv Kalangan has replaced over 50 trees since 2022.

First Edition

I dedicate this to the dreamers, healers, and givers who deliver value through art and invention, expression, and creation. With all my love.

About

In this Book I will take you through the process of becoming a fitness expert step by step. You will learn everything you need to know about the fundamentals of good training programs and how to design your very own for you or your clients.

Researching and gathering all the knowledge you need to coach others takes a lot of time, so I created this Book as a complete program to teach you everything there is to know about the three pillars of a good fitness workout.

This Book will give you all the tools you need to help others achieve their fitness goals, be it to build muscle, lose fat or simply live a more active life. If you want to build up your online fitness coaching business, be it online or in person it's important you equip yourself with the knowledge of how to correctly work with your students and understand their pain points.

The fitness coach Book is designed to develop both your personal and professional life. That means it's not just for professionals but also for beginners who want to improve their own fitness level. You don't have to have to be a personal fitness trainer or have any students yet and all you need is an interest in fitness to get started.

Why Are You Fat

Hi, today, I'll talk about a fat shredding diet secret, but before I begin, let me ask you a question. Have you ever asked yourself, why are you fat? Every time you look into the mirror wondering why people out there are having a nice summer body with full confidence while you're still struggling with your recently sized up t shirt, you might even be wondering, are you going to be like them one day? Are there any chances for you to change? Well, Of course there are. However, some bodies don't come with ease. People spend time and effort to make themselves look good. But what's important is that you're healthy from the inside out.

When I say fat burn, the first thing that comes into your mind will be exercise. Yes, Of course you need to exercise to have a nice summer body. But do you know that our eating habit affects our body the most? Having an unhealthy lifestyle not only slows down your metabolism, but also brings you chronic diseases. With a slow metabolic system, you can even gain weight by only drinking water. This is also the reason why some people slim down at a very slow rate but gain all the way back in one night. Slimming down is good, but slimming down healthily is the key point here. We want you to look into your health first instead of focusing on how you're going to slim down.

Now let's talk about the fat shredding diet secret. We all know that our bodies need a certain amount of fat for optimal functioning, but we need to know what are the right kinds of fat to consume in moderation. Some fats should be avoided at all costs, but some fats are actually good for you. Bad fats increase cholesterol and risk of diseases, but good fats protect your heart and are essential to your physical and emotional health. But the question is, how do you identify which is which? So let's learn about fats. Basically, there are two groups of fats, saturated fats and unsaturated fats, and within each group are more types of fats. Unsaturated fats are the good fats. They include polyunsaturated fatty acids and monounsaturated fats.

These fats can help lower your cholesterol levels and reduce your risk of heart disease if you learn to eat them in moderation and replacement of saturated or trans fats. Polyunsaturated fats are mostly found in vegetable oils, omega three and fatty fish and walnuts are really beneficial to health. It helps lower both blood cholesterol level and decrease cardiovascular disease. Monounsaturated fats are a good source of antioxidant vitamin E. These types of fats are typically liquid at room temperature, but solidify if refrigerated olive oil is a great choice. Mediterranean countries consume lots of it as its dietary component is credited with the low levels of heart disease in those countries.

Saturated fats are the bad fats found in animal products and in vegetable fats that are liquid at room temperature such as coconut and palm. Saturated fats are bad. If consumed on a large scale, you should keep it under 10 percent of your total calories. Let's talk about the evil fats here. We've been hearing a lot about trans fatty acids or trans fats. These days, trans fats are even more dangerous than saturated fats. These evil fats have absolutely no positive benefit to the human body in any way. Yet they've been scientifically proven to harm the body.

In many ways, trans fats can increase your bad or LDL cholesterol levels lower your good or HDL cholesterol levels cause heart disease, strokes and diabetes. Artificial trans fats are extensively used in frying baked goods like cookies, crackers, icings, packaged snacks and certain margarines. You're probably consuming trans fats on a daily basis, considering the fact that it's unanimously agreed upon by everyone in the nutrition field that trans fats are really bad for your health. You should either consume minimal trans fats in your diet or pretty much avoid them completely for best results. Now that you've learned about fats, it's time to learn how to design your own diet to shed those extra pounds.

Creating a weight loss diet that caters to your own taste preferences is the golden rule to a successful diet plan. Don't go for an extreme diet plan just because you're desperate for a drastic change in your weight. It's unrealistic, and you rarely get to your goal. Ideally, small changes in a healthy direction over time works magic on your body. Follow these simple, magical steps to creating your own fat shredding diet. Identify your current diet. Keep a careful diary log of your normal food intake for seven days. Eat as per usual. But keep a record of what you have consumed each day. How much at each meal or snack.

For example, how many bowls of cereal? One or two. How much milk, what type of milk. And then you calculate the amount of calories you intake for each meal, add all seven days, total calories intake and divide by seven. This will give you a good idea of the caloric intake you're currently consuming at your current body weight design. A new diet, dream big but start small, be realistic and take small steps towards big success. A safe weight loss that will most likely be permanently consistent is one pound a week. Do your math. One pound is equal to three thousand five hundred calories. Three thousand five hundred divided by seven days a week equals five hundred calories each day. Identify your daily average calorie count and subtract 500 calories.

However, keep in mind that you should not lower your calorie intake to less than one thousand five hundred without advice from a professional registered dietitian. Play of substitution. Don't quit eating. Learn to substitute healthier foods that you like and reduce portions of high calorie foods that you like so you can achieve the new lower daily calorie count. Let's just say you love burgers and almost can't live without them. It's OK, eat a burger. But instead of eating the whole thing, as is lower calorie count, by cutting the portion size or substituting a certain ingredient, eat half of it rather than the whole opt for lean chicken meat rather than fattening beef patty, a sprinkle of chili flakes instead of using chili sauce. The easiest and most possible way to achieve huge calorie savings is by changing the way your favorite foods are prepared.

Avoid frying and rich or thick sauces. Opt for steam, bake, broil, roast or even better, just eat it fresh. Next, I would like to share with you the secret to staying full. Are you always hungry? Do you eat more than three meals a day but still feel hungry all the time? Have you ever wondered why the secret is to reach for foods that satisfy your tummy instead of ones that only cater to your appetite but leave you hungry for more? In a study published in the American Journal of Clinical Nutrition, researchers found that some high calorie foods like bakery treats not only don't make you full, but they actually trigger your appetite.

In the research experiment, participants who are fed a meal of such foods actually ended up eating twice as much over the rest of the day, 3000 calories in all as compared to those participants fed a low fat and low calorie meal. Now, here's the deal. Find fit or fast food? Look for low fat, low calorie and fulfilling options. Brown rice, grilled, skinless, lean meat, whole wheat bread salads. They're extremely filling, actually, soup. And best yet, plain water goes along with any meal and you'll feel full for sure. So that's it. The ultimate secret to a fat shredding diet. Learn about your food, eat smart, and you'll be shedding those fats away with not just a healthy body, but also a happy tummy.

Fat Burn Mantra

In this chapter, we'll talk about the fat burn mantra and how to eat like a celebrity and not get fat. Believe it or not, it's all about the mindset. If your body is a car, your mind is the engine, your mindset drives your body. It fuels your will and determination to work towards your goal. It can be difficult to achieve and maintain your ideal body shape and weight. It takes more than just healthy eating and regular exercise. A positive and motivated mindset is essential to keep going if you tell yourself negative things. This is so hard. I can't do this. You're not going to make it far. But if you encourage yourself with thoughts like I can do this, nothing can stop me. I'm going to lose five pounds by the end of the week. You're motivated to achieve your diet goals, mindsets or assumptions or beliefs that you established to govern your behavior and choices.

There are two types of mindsets: fixed and growth oriented people with a fixed mindset. Think of the absolutes and allow little to no room for possibilities. They're fixated to their definite opinion and would not budge from that framed mindset when faced with a challenge, they tend to take the easy way out to avoid failure and embarrassment. This is a psychological principle known as self handicapping. People with a growth mindset strongly believe in possibilities. They're open minded, willing to adopt new ideas and learn to improve. They take on challenges even at the risk of failing. They're open to embrace failure because they know they can learn from it to successfully shed fat.

First, shed your negative thinking. Research shows that one of the many important factors that influences weight loss is your attitude, whether or not you believe you can do it. And if it is worth doing, it's a simple theory that you think will affect how you feel and in turn the actions you take, similar to how conventional medications often treat symptoms of disease without addressing the cause. Weight loss diets often address your weight without addressing what has led you to be overweight. Being overweight is not as simple as eating too much or moving too little. There's an underlying combination of subconscious conditioning, self-worth issues, emotional difficulties and more.

You might be able to lose a couple of pounds by slowly changing your diet and doing exercises, but it won't last long. Specific diets will only be temporarily effective. Addressing the underlying psychological cause that led you to be overweight while applying a balanced diet and exercise will ensure you long lasting weight loss. Follow these life changing mantras that could help you eliminate any sort of destructive thoughts that sabotage your body weight. Others opinions don't matter. As long as I love my body, I will eliminate the fear of others' opinions. When we despise how we look and how we feel, our bodies reflect and adopt these ideas due to the environmental conditioning.

Many people think they must be thin to really love themselves. It's all because of others' opinions. But loving yourself must come first for your weight loss efforts to be effective. Shed your fears, learn to love your own body and each small change that occurs to it through your dieting effort. Slow and steady learn as you go. If you lose your fats too fast, it may not last a little. Goes a long way. Focus on progress over perfection because no perfection comes along without long term progression. Be patient and work with a well planned diet for the long run. Your body takes time to adjust to all the changes. A diet done in the right way will ensure that your body will be accustomed to the changes and that the effects are definitely longer lasting.

I may not be where I want to be, but I'm better than where I was. I don't have enough time. Fifteen minutes. A workout won't make a difference. Sound familiar? This is the kind of statement that gives you permission to veer from the healthy habits that help you lose weight. Don't find excuses. A tiny effort done is always better than none. Fifteen minutes each day, rather than none at all, is still going to make a change to your body, regardless of how significant it is. Always remember that every small step taken is a step closer to your goal. Never underestimate yourself.

Now I'll share with you how to eat like a celebrity and not get fat. When you see photos of Rihanna's slim but glamorous silhouette or Jessica Alba's flat post pregnancy tummy, you'll probably wonder how celebrities stay so lean and how they always managed to snap back into shape in the blink of an eye. Truth is, some celebrities go to strange and outrageous lengths to get or stay thin, even though most of them swear that they're perfect. Bodies come from exercising and eating clean. It's risky to just blindly follow those alleged diet plans of celebrities. But fret not, because here's some legit, useful and healthy tips quoted directly from A-list celebrity trainers.

You could steal and not be wary of the risk tips from celebrity trainers. No. One, celebrities eat breakfast. Number two, they pick their veggies. Three, they snack on healthy snacks, Of course. And number four, they don't stop drinking water. Now, let's talk about the first tip. Celebrities eat breakfast. We all know. The importance of breakfast, but there are still many people skipping their breakfast on a daily basis. Celebrity trainer Gunnar Peterson, trainer to Jennifer Lopez, Penelope Cruz, Leah Remini introduced the idea of eating within 30 minutes of waking up in the morning. You want to send your body a signal that you're not starving, so it starts burning fat, says Peterson. Tripe, oatmeal, scrambled egg, whites, fruits. These ingredients provide filling fiber, protein and vitamins.

Research shows that breakfast eaters are more successful at long term weight loss as it helps jumpstart your metabolism and prevents overeating throughout the day. Here's a tip to be picky in choosing your veggies. No, celebrities don't plan and pick their own veggies. They're taught by their trainers to be picky and what veggies they eat. Here's a tip to slimming down a few inches for a seen event. Nutritionist Keri Wyatt made famous singer Fergie stock up on water, veggies and fruits, lettuce, celery, cucumbers, watermelon grapes to help get rid of bloating as those veggies work by flushing out your system, cauliflower, broccoli, cabbage and pears lead to gas and bloating. So if you'd like to be seen, lean for the night.

Remember to avoid these right before an event. Tip number three, they snack healthy snacks, Of course. Trainer Valerie Waters had her clients, Jennifer Garner, Elizabeth Berkley, carry one hundred and fifty calorie snacks wherever they go.

A few all time favorite snack combos include apple slices with low fat string cheese, a couple of crackers topped with chicken salad or a few slices of turkey ham with fruits. According to Valerie Waters, it's important to eat something every three to four hours because you can go from feeling kind of hungry to thinking you're starving badly if your blood sugar can drop quickly.

Healthy snacking helps curb your cravings and gives you an instant energy boost to keep you satiated. Tip number four, they don't stop drinking. I hope you're not thinking about alcohol. Drink water. Of course it's water. They never stop drinking water. Celebrity trainer and nutritionist Harley Pasternak, whose clients include Lady Gaga, Rihanna, Megan Fox, Robert Downey Jr., urges the importance of hydration. According to Pasternack, thirst can often be mistaken for hunger, so regularly sipping water throughout the day can keep excess calories off your plate and your mouth. Now that you already know the four tips from celebrity trainers, let's move on to the three famous celebrity diet plans. The first one is the five factor diet created by nutritionist and celebrity fitness guru Harley Pasternak.

The five factors consist of the elements. Each meal should include protein, complex carbs, fats, fibers and fluids. This diet plan requires you to eat five meals a day with recipes of no more than five ingredients. And guess what? You get one cheat day per week where you're allowed to eat anything you'd like. Celebrities like Eva Mendez, Alicia Keys, Megan Fox and Katy Perry are the followers of this diet. The next diet plan is the Zone Diet, developed by former scientist Dr. Barry Sears. This diet involves obtaining forty percent of your daily caloric intake from carbohydrates, 30 percent from fats and 30 percent from carbs.

Sears created this diet based on balancing the correct amount of amino acids with carbs because it helps control your appetite and prevent overeating. You are to eat three portion controlled meals and two snacks a day. Famous Hollywood celebrity Jennifer Aniston was such a big fan of this diet, some even called it the Jennifer Aniston diet. And lastly, the prestigious Free Press chooses a California based company whose products are in general dense and nutrition, low and sugar, yet high in fiber and are proven to be a sensible way of consuming calories. It has been widely popular among celebrities to follow this six juices a day. Twelve hundred calorie intense cleanse. This press juice free diet is said to be a major blowout beta.

Every morning you'll receive a daily supplement of juices delivered to your doorstep. Each fresh nutrient pack drink is specially designed to replace meals and snacks, and you're highly advised to avoid alcohol, caffeine and nicotine in order to achieve a complete cleansing Hollywood celebrity. And also a busy mom, Nicole Richie, sips on these juices. I drink these between meals to be sure I'm getting everything I need. I don't go a day without greens, juice, kale, spinach, cucumber, celery and romaine. It's actually really good, says Richie Leslie. I'll share with you the star diet mantras and tricks. Now the Hollywood stars are spilling their secrets to their perfect body shape.

Aren't you excited? Nicki Minaj is secret, there is no sugar or starch. She lost ten pounds by giving up Snickers insides of potatoes three days before a big shoot. Hilary Duff's secret is simply treating yourself. She does boxing drills and runs a lot. She eats a lot of chicken, but she rewards herself to Kaley Cuoco. Secret is no alcohol. She skips alcohol for a lean body, claiming that alcohol is the body. She also works out four to five times a week. Yoga, horseback riding. Etc. Jennifer Lopez's secret is cardio all the time. She lost eight pounds by eating lean meat, broccoli and carrots. Jessica Simpson's secret is oatmeal and small portions. She eats small portions of chicken and oatmeal.

She also does strength training chapters three times a week. Miranda Lambert's secret is to have everything in moderation. She plans her daily intake if her breakfast is high in calories. She picks a low calorie dinner like grilled chicken and sweet potatoes. She still snacks on her must have snacks, Cheetos by doing daily hour long cardio drills. Ashley Tisdale's secret is again breakfast. She always starts her day with fresh fruit and egg, white omelet and whole wheat toast. And there you have it. All the secrets from top celebrities to start blasting those fats away. Hope these tips and tricks motivated you and encouraged you to start burning those fats away from your body.

Easy Fat Killer Technique

In this chapter, you'll learn about easy fat killer techniques, but before going into detail, let's talk about cardio. The word cardio is short for cardiovascular. Cardio workouts are endurance exercises that strengthen the circulatory system consisting of the heart and blood vessels in your body. People do cardio over long stretches of time as it makes the heart beat faster and pump more blood through your system. Bringing nutrients and oxygen to every cell cardio workout can simply be explained as a physical exercise of low to high intensity. That depends on the Aerobic energy generating process of the exercise you do. It's any activity that gets your heart rate raised to 50 to 75 percent of your maximum heart rate. Calculate your maximum with the Formula 220 minus your age.

For example, if you're twenty five years old, two hundred twenty minus twenty five equals one ninety five. Cardio workout burns calories in your body. Most people do cardio training to lose weight gain, body mass train stamina, etc. There are different intensities to cardio exercises. Low or moderate intensity exercise normally leaves you feeling slightly breathless but still able to comfortably talk to someone. Low intensity exercises include walking, swimming or cycling. On the other hand, high intensity exercises will leave you speaking in short sentences as you sweat and breathe rapidly. High intensity exercises include running, sprinting, aerobic classes like Zumba or circuit training. It is commonly believed that long, slow and low intensity cardio is best for fat loss as it utilizes aerobic exercises that burn fat during exercise.

While some find high intensity cardio more effective for fat loss as it burns higher amounts of overall fat. So the question is, how do you know which one is better, low intensity or high intensity? The short answer is that the best type of cardio, whether low or high intensity, is the one you will do consistently over time. The optimal plan is to start at lower intensity if you're new to cardio and slowly work your way up to higher intensities as your endurance and cardiorespiratory work capacity improve. Reason is because beginners doing high intensity training are highly prone to body burnout due to continuous hard core training that causes strains towards your body, especially your muscles and joints.

Burnout will leave you feeling extremely tired, cranky, exhausted and too worn out to stick with your routine. If you're a beginner, try interval training, warm up at a low intensity and alternate one minute of high intensity with one minute low. Or you can call it recovery intensity. As you progress, you can then start to either increase the intensity or the duration of the high intensity part or decrease the duration of the low intensity part. By doing so, you'll be able to burn more calories during the workout at higher intensity. Remember, losing fat is about burning more calories than we consume over time. Combining both Elai and HIV will contribute to hitting your weight loss goals faster. Remember to progress slowly with baby steps, though doing too much too soon can lead to injury or burnout, which can take you out of the game.

Here are the advantages of both low intensity and high intensity cardio. Maybe you should screencap this table for your future reference. It'll help you decide the best workout that suits your body best at specific stages. So now that you know the benefits of low intensity and high intensity cardio, I'll show you some examples of exercises for low intensity, moderate intensity and high intensity respectively, so that you have a rough idea for low intensity. You can briskly walk, do some stretching routines, yoga, swimming and some simple household chores, such as vacuuming, mopping yard work or washing the car for moderate intensity. You can do speed walking, cycling basically up, leveling any low intensity exercise by a natural simply work as a moderate intensity workout for high intensity.

You can do aerobics exercises, jump rope, high speed running or jogging push ups or jumping jacks. Now, I've prepared a ten minute beginner, high intensity workout. Here's a little tip for a beginner high cardio workout for you. Complete three sets of twenty seconds of work. Ten seconds of rest. First step. Jab. Cross. Front. Right side. Stand with your right foot in front of the left. Hips facing your left side. Bring your arms up into a boxing position. Jab or punch. Forward with the right arm, then throw a cross punch with the left arm, letting your body rotate as your left arm crosses over your body to the right. Your body weight should be over your right foot with your back heel picking up off the floor slightly.

Bring both arms back into your body, shifting your weight back to the starting position and facing front. This is the front move repeated on the left side. Second step jab. Cross front, left side, third step. Jumping jacks start by standing upright with your feet at hip width apart and your arms at your sides. Jump your feet out while raising your arms. As fast as possible, if a regular jumping jack is too difficult, step side to side while raising your arms instead. Fourth step, sumo squats position your feet a little more than hip width apart and pointing your toes out at a 45 degree angle, keeping your weight in your heels back flat and chest upright.

Lower yourself until your thighs are parallel to the floor. Engage your glutes and quads and push back to the start position. Repeat, cool down with an overhead stretch, reverse, lunge and forward fold. All you have to do is follow the killer cardio plan. Using this workout schedule is a framework you can easily add in any cardio exercise that falls into the corresponding workout style.

Yo-Yo Effect

Have you ever seen some weight loss TV program where some contestants lose a big amount of weight only to gain it back almost right away? Ever wondered how and why that happened? It's all because of the Yo-Yo effect. What's the Yo-Yo Effect? Yo-Yo Effect, also known as weight cycling, is the cyclical loss and gain of weight resembling the up and down motion of a Yo-Yo losing weight quickly by doing a diet plan, then regaining it, falling back into your eating habits, or failing to stick to your exercise routine, which leads you towards the Yo-Yo Effect. A classic Yo-Yo Dieter's weight goes up and down, but rarely stays in one place for long. People who do diets without consistency tend to fall into a vicious circle after each weight loss.

The weight gain that follows is worse than the previous one, which then makes them diet even more severely than last time. Such a Yo-Yo Effect can lead you to put on more than 20 times your normal weight or in the worst case, obesity. So what are the causes? No. One, two difficult diets, a diet plan that is too restrictive to follow over a long period of time. No, to overexerted exercises. This causes burnout and difficulty to keep it up in the long run. Number three, unbalanced diet. The same nutritional mistakes will be reproduced a few weeks or months later. Number four, extreme dieting.

This causes depression and fatigue, resulting in difficulty to sustain the willpower to continue the common reasons of yo yo dieting. Seen above are what drive yo yo dieters to eating more than they would have before dieting, causing them to rapidly regain weight. When psychological factors kick in, it's almost impossible for dieters to sustain their willpower. Therefore, old eating habits and lack of exercise caused fat and weight to bounce back as much or even more. The yo yo effect is dangerous. Why? Because the regained weight is increasingly difficult to lose. Imagine you're struggling to lose ten pounds and now you have to lose twenty pounds.

Due to the rebounding weight, anyone will go crazy. Rebounding occurs because our body remembers the effects of deprivation caused by secessions of diets over a long period of time, therefore resulting in storing more fats in reserve to prepare for future diets. It is a progressive development of obesity. Your weight will bounce back in an extreme manner, and the recovering process is twice as difficult as the previous diet process. You'll feel out of control and lose grasp on the long run, thus resulting in a rocketing weight gain leading to obesity. Besides, emotional distress leads to depressive disorders.

The suppression from previous extreme diets are bound to cause you depressive disorders like insomnia, depression, dysthymia, bipolar. Such disorders will interfere with your daily life, affecting your normal functioning and causing pain to you and your loved ones. Thus, you'll have a higher possibility of having high blood pressure, high cholesterol, gallbladder disease or cardiovascular disease, arthritis, infarction, etc.. Inconsistent food intake, unbalanced nutrition on and off extreme exercise workouts and emotional instability will eventually drive your body haywire. Your body won't be able to familiarize itself with all the changes done within an inconsistent time frame and manner.

All of the above dangers will eventually lead to the possibility of a shortened lifespan. There's nothing wrong with being ambitious and eager to achieve your ideal weight. Having the desire and the drive to meet your goal is half the battle and getting there. Be flexible and learn from your mistakes. If you try an exercise regimen or a new food plan that you don't enjoy or find hard to sustain, then try something else. Bear in mind that your goal should not be to lose as much weight as you can or as quickly as you can. You need to establish healthy patterns of eating and exercise that will help you lose weight while at the same time having long sustainability. You need to realize that trying to do too much too quickly could be your undoing.

Be realistic on the amount of changes you're able to make at once. Keep track of your progress and find sources of support as it'll be helpful for you to overcome difficulties. Exercise buddies are great and some people find a lot of value in the support they get through online communities. The most crucially essential factor in solving the yo-yo dilemma has to do with changing your behavior and practicing eating smaller, more frequent meals. Plan your food intake including hunger, fighting protein at each meal and snack plan ahead. Keep track, enlist, help. A quick sprint might get you to the finish line if you're lucky, but chances are you're going to be left exhausted and out of the game when it comes to successful weight loss. Slow and steady definitely wins the race.

Easy Yoga Practice

In this chapter, you'll learn about easy yoga practice, yoga is an ancient Indian philosophy that dates back thousands of years. It was designed as a path to spiritual enlightenment. But in modern times, the physical aspects of Hatti yoga have found huge popularity as a gentle form of exercise and stress management. There are many different varieties of yoga, but each one essentially relies on structured poses. Astana practiced with breath awareness. Researchers have discovered that the regular practice of yoga may produce many health benefits, including fitness and normalization of blood pressure. Yoga is a renowned antidote to stress.

Over time, yoga practitioners report lower levels of stress and increased feelings of happiness and well-being. This is because concentrating on the postures and the breath acts as a powerful form of meditation. If you can breathe, you can do yoga wellknown, a Iyengar teacher, Patricia Walden, once said. Hence, yoga is becoming so popular today. Do you know what the biggest benefits of yoga are? No one improved strength, routine and consistent practice of the various yoga asanas has helped people to build strength and improve lean muscle mass, most notably with respect to several muscle groups underutilized and chosen athletic disciplines of swimming, cycling and running.

These gains have enhanced core body stability and significantly impeded overuse injury by strengthening the supportive but otherwise underdeveloped muscles surrounding the more utilized muscles, creating a more balanced and optimally functional overall strength number to balance through a consistent yoga practice, you'll notice that your coordination and balance have improved immensely. Why is this important? Better balance and coordination means enhanced control over how you move your body, which in turn leads to better technique and form number three flexibility. Yoga invariably improves joint and muscular flexibility, which is crucial to the body's overall structural soundness.

Enhanced joint and muscle appliance translates to a greater range of motion or an increase in the performance latitude for a particular movement or series of movements. For example, a swimmer with supple shoulder and hip joints is able to capture and pull more water than a swimmer with a more limited range of motion. The result is more forward movement per stroke as well as enhanced muscular economy. In turn, this increased range of motion provides a greater ability to strength conditioning a particular muscle group due to the amelioration and overall force that can be exerted with each movement number for free. Your mind.

The ability to create a stress free mind is a significant benefit of yoga practice. Physical practice is used as a tool to enhance breath control, which helps improve focus and concentration, allowing clarity of thought and clear decision making. It is a valuable tool in any sporting arena. Mental practice in any sport will teach you how to gain control of your emotional state. So arousal levels and anxiety don't impede your performance. Number five reduces anxiety and stress. Yoga helps you reduce cortical levels and increase calming hormones, improve cognitive function, reduce blood pressure and heart rate, and increase immune function.

These benefits combine to allow for better rest, sleep and recovery, as well as provide the ability to think more clearly under pressure. Here are three tips for yoga practice. Number one, side effects and risk number two things to consider. Number three, training, licensing and certification. Let's talk about the side effects and risks of yoga practice. We all know that yoga is generally low impact and safe for healthy people when practiced appropriately under the guidance of a well-trained instructor. Overall, those who practice yoga have a low rate of side effects, and the risk of serious injury from yoga is quite low. However, certain types of strokes, as well as pain from nerve damage, are among the rare possible side effects of practicing yoga.

However, women who are pregnant and people with certain medical conditions such as hypertension, heart attack or asthma should modify or avoid some yoga poses. Here are some things to consider when you've decided to practice yoga. If you're considering practicing yoga, do not use yoga to replace conventional medical care or to postpone seeing a health care provider about pain or any other medical condition. If you have a medical condition, talk to your health care provider. Before starting yoga, you should ask a trusted source to recommend a yoga practitioner to find out the training and experience of any practitioner you were considering.

Besides, you need to know that everybody's body is different and yoga posture should be modified based on individual abilities. Carefully selecting an instructor who is experienced with and attentive to your needs is an important step forward in helping you practice yoga safely. Ask about the physical demands of the type of yoga in which you are interested and inform your yoga instructor about any medical condition you have. Carefully think about the type of yoga you're interested in. For example, hot yoga such as Bikram yoga may involve standing and moving in. Human environments with temperatures as high as 105 degrees Fahrenheit, because such settings may be physically stressful.

People who practice hot yoga should take certain precautions. These include drinking water before, during and after a hot yoga practice and wearing suitable clothing. People with conditions that may be affected by excessive heat, such as heart disease, lung disease and a prior history of heat stroke may want to avoid this form of yoga altogether. Women who are pregnant may want to check with their health care providers before starting hot yoga. There are many training programs for yoga teachers throughout the country. These programs range from a few days to more than two years.

Standards for teacher training and certification differ depending on the style of yoga. There are organizations that register yoga teachers and training programs that have complied with a certain curriculum and educational standards. For example, one nonprofit group, the Yoga Alliance, requires at least 200 hours of training with a specified number of hours in areas including techniques, training, methodology, anatomy, physiology and philosophy. Most yoga therapists training programs involve 500 hours or more. The International

Association of Yoga Therapists is developing standards for yoga therapy training. Next, I'll share with you the eight different types of yoga moves for beginners.

We have the warrior pose, tree, pose, triangle, pose seated, twist upward facing dog pose, pigeon pose, crow pose and child's pose. And here's how you do the warrior pose. First stand with your legs three to four feet apart. Turn out your right foot ninety degrees and your left foot slightly keeping your shoulders down. Extend your arms to the sides with your palms down. Lunge into your right knee at ninety degrees. Keep your knee over your foot and don't let it go past your toes. Aim your focus over your hand for as long as you like. Then switch sides when doing the tree pose.

Begin with the mountain pose, then shift your weight onto your left leg, keeping your hips facing forward. Place the sole of your right foot inside your left thigh and find your balance when you're there. Take a prayer position with your hands to kick it up a notch. Reach your arms up as you would in a mountain pose. Be sure to repeat on the other side for the triangle pose. Take the warrior pose on your right side without lunging into your knee. Then touch the inside of your right foot with the outside of your right hand. Reach up to the ceiling with your left hand. Turn your gaze toward and past your left hand to stretch your back. Don't forget to repeat it on the other side. Four seated twist. First, sit on the floor and extend your legs.

Cross your right foot over the outside of your left thigh, bend your left knee, keeping your right knee pointed towards the ceiling. Keep your right hand on the floor behind you to stay stable and place your left elbow to the outside of your right knee. Twist to the right as far as you can, moving from your abdomen. Be sure to keep both sides of your butt on the floor. Do this on both sides when doing the upward facing dog pose first lay face down on the floor with your thumbs under your shoulders and your legs extended with the tops of your feet on the floor. Tuck your hips downward as you squeeze your glutes, keeping your shoulders down, push up and lift your chest off the ground, relax and repeat.

As for the pigeon pose, start in a push up position, palms under your shoulders, place your left knee on the floor near your shoulders with your left heel by your right hip. Press your hands to the floor and sit back with your chest lifted. You can also lower your chest closer to the floor for a stretch. Try it on the other side for the crockpots, get into downward facing dog position, then walk your feet forward until your knees touch your arms carefully. Bend your elbows and lift your heels off the floor. Rest your knees against the outside of your upper arms. Keep your abs engaged and legs pressed against your arms. You can leave your toes on the floor or if you approach, lift them off and hover.

To do this, try to keep tuck tight with your heels close to your butt. When you're ready, push your upper arms against your shins and draw your inner groin deep into the pelvis to help you with the lift. When doing the child pose, sit upright comfortably on your heels, roll your torso forward and bring your forehead to rest on the ground in front of you, extend your arms forward, lower your chest to your knees as close as you comfortably can. Hold the pose and breathe into your torso. Exhale and release to get deeper into your fold. And there you have it. A simple to follow step by step guide for beginner yoga poses.

List of Fat-Pumping Foods To Avoid

With so much talk of healthy foods and what you should be eating, the foods that are the worst for us can get overlooked. The reason it's so hard to avoid these kinds of foods is because the things that make them bad also make them taste good. Fatty foods typically taste good. So do sweet and salty ones, which means a lot of the foods you love are likely not the best things you can have, but you don't have to resort to living like Tom Hanks in Castaway. There are plenty of foods that you can turn to taste amazing and won't jeopardize your well-being. It's about learning why certain foods are bad so you can make better choices on a day to day basis.

That being said, here are some dietary landmines to watch out for and step around. A new study published in the journal Preventing Chronic Disease revealed that 84 percent of packaged foods that listed zero grams trans fat on their nutrition facts label still had partially hydrogenated oil, the main dietary source of trans fat in the ingredient list. Current laws allow companies to round down fewer than five grams of trans fat per serving to zero. The good news is the amount of trans fat we eat has dropped in the past 30 years, according to a recent study published in the Journal of the American Heart Association.

Men are consuming 32 percent less trans fat and women 35 percent less than they were in 1980. Still, one point nine percent of men's daily calories and one point seven percent of women's daily calories come from trans fat. Today, the

American Heart Association recommends limiting trans fat to no more than one percent of total calories consumed. Even a few daily grams of these fats increase bad cholesterol, decrease good cholesterol and clog arteries. And Harvard researchers estimate that trans fats cause up to 200 28000 cases of heart disease and 50000 deaths annually. Since two grams is the most you should have in a day allowing food with point five grams or less to call themselves trans fat free. It's a real problem.

Simply said, you're best off avoiding trans fat containing foods completely. I'll also show you some quick examples of food rich and trans fat that you might not even be aware of. The first is a non-dairy coffee creamer. Half a gram of trans fat and creamer can quickly turn into multiple, since consumers tend to use more than the serving size of a teaspoon per cup. And the typical American coffee drinker guzzles an average of three cups of Joe per day. On many zero trans fat labels, you can find partially hydrogenated oils as the second or third ingredient listed. The second one is peanut butter. Some companies use partially hydrogenated oils to achieve a long shelf life and creamy texture. So check the label to be safe. Opt for the natural variety.

Although it's chunkier, it's also healthier and normally made with just salt and peanuts, not oils loaded with trans fat. You might think that avoiding usual pizza is good, but frozen pizza is equally bad. Trans fat sneaks into the dough of many frozen pizzas with about point three grams and just one slice. San Diego mother of two, Katie Simpson, sued Nestle for five million dollars last year over the use of trans fat in its frozen pizzas sold by DiGiorgio Stuffers in California Pizza Kitchen.

The case was dismissed since she knowingly purchased and consumed the pizza. One solution is to make your own pie at home. Popcorn is unhealthy as well. I know it's your Friday night movie staple, but microwavable popcorn puts the spotlight on trans fats.

The true culprits are the toppings. Butter flavoring can include five grams of trans fat per serving, while caramel flavoring can contain as many as one point five grams. Some extra buttery varieties can have up to fifteen grams of trans fats per bag, which is all too easy to inhale in one sitting. Stay away from the microwave popcorn, says Napoli. Just do the old fashioned air popper use an actual oil to pop the kernels in? You might love them, but packaged cookies are the devil's. Even the beloved Girl Scout cookies still sneak some trans fat in, despite a label that says trans fat free.

You may be able to justify those because they only happen a few times a year. But check to see if your favorite store bought it. Cookies are made with partially hydrogenated cooking oils. Chances are they are including Chips Ahoy and Keibler, although some brands like Oreos now use high olive oils instead so they can provide shelf stable cookies at a reasonable cost. Lastly, margarine margarine consumption boomed during the butter shortages of World War Two, with even Eleanor Roosevelt promoting it as her toast topping of choice. But it's a recipe for trans fat overload to create the creamy spread. Liquid vegetable oils are blasted with hydrogen.

The more solid the margarine, the more it's been hydrogenated. Many labels claim to have zero grams of trans fat, but the label lists partially hydrogenated oils. Those small amounts of trans fat can add up when you slather margarine on your food. High fructose corn syrup, or HFS, is an ingredient that didn't exist before 1960, but has a strong appeal to food manufacturers because it's so very sweet, cheap to make and easy to store. According to Davidsen Zenko, in the ABS diet, the human body doesn't have a shutoff switch for HFS the way it does with real sugar. This leads us to keep drinking a cola or eating sweet treats long after we would have stopped if they were naturally sweetened.

Those who pay attention to what they eat may have noticed high fructose corn syrup creeping into an alarming number of foods in the supermarket aisle. Corn subsidies and other trends have pushed this relatively unhealthy substance into many of the general food groups that we shop for on a regular basis. Here are some of the popular food and drink items that contain high fructose corn syrup, an element with a lot of sugar that has been known to contribute to diabetes and other conditions when eating in excess soft drinks are packed with HFS. It's no surprise to most of us that soda is chock full of high fructose corn syrup.

To those who aren't used to the drink, that stuff can be almost sickeningly sweet. Even diet varieties can have a large amount of this sweetener, added to the fact that soda machines can be found on the street corner in the lobbies of buildings and in almost any public space. And it's easy to see why obesity and sugar related conditions are such a problem in today's world. Also, sauces and salad dressing will hurt your waistline. Most ketchup ends up on French fries, and few stopped to consider that it's actually acting to make the fries unhealthier. That's because it uses high fructose corn syrup as its number three ingredient, at least in a bottle of America's number one best selling ketchup.

Heinz, there's four grams of total sugar and the majority of that will come from HFS. You might think yogurt is good, but you're dead wrong. Although many dieters add yogurt to their daily menu, they'd better watch out for what it contains with many of the brands using high fructose corn syrup to make them taste good. Going with a light version of yogurt no doubt means you're getting an artificial sweetener, which can be just as bad. Pay extra attention to processed snacks, too. There are other items that the average consumer wouldn't think of as HFS candidates look at the labels for things like breaded meats or processed potato items and make sure that the sweetener is not lurking somewhere on that label. Monosodium glutamate, also known as MSG, is a commonly used food enhancer whose taste is described as umami.

Like taste is usually divided into four categories. Sweet, salty, sour and bitter glutamate is said to have a fifth unique taste called umami, which is described as the savory flavor of meats. MSG is used to enhance this so-called umami flavor and is known to have negative side effects even when ingested in small amounts. Since MSG is found so frequently in processed foods, it is very hard to avoid, except in cases when the packaging specifically states that the product contains no MSG. Even then, manufactured free glutamic acid can be found in different forms such as , yeast, MSG, Tawila, yeast, yeast extracts and the hydrolyzed proteins can raise levels of glutamate, which in turn stimulates neurons synthetically. Glutamates may have different names, but are all essentially MSG.

Some common glutamate strongly related to MSG include hydrolyzed proteins, elderlies, yeasts, protein concentrates, yeast extract, glutamic acid and the list goes on. These glutamates can be found in very common grocery items such as low fat yogurt, canned soups, chips and most ranch and cheese flavored foods. In a 2014 study published in Life Science, researchers found that young rats treated with MSG were more susceptible to developing anxiety and depressive behaviors. Examples of food rich and MSG are vegan breakfast, sausage, bacon bits, veggie burger and nuggets and fried food. Walk into any big grocery store and you'll find that artificial sweeteners are everywhere.

They're tucked into soft drinks, baked goods and fruit juices to make them taste sweet without the extra calories. Most products that contain artificial sweeteners are usually labeled as diet or reduced sugar, but not all are. You can even find some in foods that claim to have natural ingredients because they're not always clearly labeled on food packaging. Consumers may not realize that they're eating them. Artificial sweeteners have been under the spotlight for decades now as health food advocates point out that they come with a list of side effects, much like a drug. The side effects that are claimed by those against sweeteners like aspartame include some really severe conditions such as depression, insomnia, blindness, tinnitus, hives and a contributing factor to things like Alzheimer's and PMS.

Examples of foods rich and artificial sweeteners are light food and beverages with the word light or low sugar, Diet Coke and packaged snacks. High levels of sodium or salt can really wreak havoc on your body. Not only does it cause you to retain water, but it also increases blood pressure and can lead to complications with the heart. Almost all heart patients are put on a low sodium diet. Whether they suffered a heart attack, stroke or are at risk for them. It makes sense to watch your sodium levels long before it reaches the point of a doctor telling you to do so or forcing you onto a diet to help save your life. Foods high in sodium. Ah, cheese, salty snacks, frozen meals, bread and tortillas, foods high in calories can really add to your waistline in a hurry if you're not careful.

The reason they're so sneaky is because you can consume hundreds of calories quickly and not even be aware of it. A popular dieting theory is that the fewer calories taken in, the more weight you'll lose, all else being equal. That's why you see people going on low calorie diets and trying to burn calories in the gym. You don't have to go to extremes, but finding the calories you consume will lead to a healthier you. Examples of food choices high in calories are pasta dishes, chocolate and chia seeds. It's not as if you have to go low carb, no carb, but you should still keep an eye on your carbohydrate intake. In fact, there's even a recommended daily allowance set at one hundred and thirty grams.

Why are there so many carbs? Unhealthy foods high in carbohydrates will be digested quickly and tend to increase your blood sugar levels. This causes a release of insulin which produces glycogen which gets stored in the body as fat. They're also responsible for making you feel hungry again quickly and can lead to more eating and overeating than would otherwise happen. Examples are bagels, coffee, drinks and movie popcorn.

Fat Burn Supplement & Detox Plan

In this chapter, we'll talk about fat burn supplements and detox plans. The majority of adults in the United States take one or more dietary supplements either every day or occasionally. Today's dietary supplements include vitamins, minerals, herbs and botanicals, amino acids, enzymes and many other products. Dietary supplements come in a variety of forms, traditional tablets, capsules and powders, as well as drinks and energy bars. Popular supplements include vitamin D and E minerals like calcium and iron herbs such as echinacea and garlic, and specialty products like glucosamine, probiotics and fish oils. The pursuit of health has never been more informed. We know more about the fields of medicine and nutrition than ever.

Technological advances now allow scientists and clinicians to predict one susceptibility to certain diseases or conditions by analyzing the DNA in cells obtained from a cheek swab. We know that the conditions of fetuses exposed to in utero can influence the risk of disease in adulthood. We've come so far in understanding the biology of our bodies, in the biochemistry of the nutrients and other substances we ingest. The United States is recognized among the leaders of the world in technology and medicine. And yet, despite all these advances, Americans are unhealthier, more overweight or obese, more prone to chronic disease than ever.

Where did we go wrong? All products labeled as a dietary supplement KARIUS Supplement Facts panel that lists the contents amount of active ingredients per serving and other added ingredients like fillers, binders and flavorings. The manufacturer suggests the serving size, but you or your health care provider might decide that a different amount is more appropriate for you. However, there are things that you really need to know before you start consuming it. Number one, effectiveness. Number two, safety and risk. And number three, quality. Number one, effectiveness. If you don't eat a nutritious variety of foods, some supplements might help you get adequate amounts of essential nutrients.

However, supplements can't take the place of the variety of foods that are important to a healthy diet. Scientific evidence shows that some dietary supplements are beneficial for overall health and for managing some health conditions. For example, calcium and vitamin D are important for keeping bones strong and reducing bone loss. Folic acid decreases the risk of certain birth defects, and omega three fatty acids from fish oils might help. Some people with heart disease or other supplements need more study to determine their value. The U.S. Food and Drug Administration, or FDA, does not determine whether dietary supplements are effective before they are marketed.

Number two, safety and risk. Many supplements contain active ingredients that can have strong effects in the body. Always be alert to the possibility of unexpected side effects, especially when taking a new product. Supplements are most likely to cause side effects or harm when people take them instead of prescribed medicines or when people take many supplements in combination, some supplements can increase the risk of bleeding. Or if a person takes them before or after surgery, they can affect the person's response to anesthesia. Dietary supplements can also interact with certain prescription drugs in ways that might cause problems. Here's some examples.

For your reference, vitamin K can reduce the ability of the blood thinner Coumadin to prevent blood from clotting. St. John's Wort can speed the breakdown of many drugs, including antidepressants and birth control pills, and thereby reduce these drugs effectiveness. Antioxidant supplements like vitamin C and E might reduce the effectiveness of some types of cancer chemotherapy. Keep in mind that some ingredients found in dietary supplements are added to a growing number of foods, including breakfast cereals and beverages. As a result, you may be getting more of these ingredients than you think, and more might not be better.

Taking more than you need is always more expensive and can also raise your risk of experiencing side effects. For example, getting too much vitamin A can cause headaches and liver damage, reduce bone strength and cause birth defects. Excess iron causes nausea and vomiting and may damage the liver and other organs. Be cautious about taking dietary supplements if you're pregnant or nursing. Also, be careful about giving them beyond a basic multivitamin or mineral product to a child. Most dietary supplements have not been well tested for safety and pregnant women, nursing mothers or children.

Number three, quality dietary supplements are complex products. The FDA has established quality standards for dietary supplements to help ensure their identity, purity, strength and composition. These standards are designed to prevent the inclusion of the wrong ingredient, the addition of too much or too little of an ingredient, the possibility of contamination and the improper packaging and labeling of a product. The FDA periodically inspects facilities that manufacture dietary supplements. In addition, several independent organizations offer quality testing and allow products that pass these tests to display their seal of approval. These seals of approval provide assurance that the product was.

Properly manufactured contains the ingredients listed on the label and does not contain harmful levels of contaminants, these seals of approval do not guarantee that a product is safe or effective. Organizations that offer this quality testing include U.S. Pharmacopeia, Consumer Lab, Dotcom and NSF International. For much of the 20th century, nutrition research focused largely on the health risks and benefits of single nutrients. The findings translated into public health messages telling us to reduce fat, limit cholesterol, increase fiber, get more calcium, take vitamins E, C and D and so on.

But as scientists learn more, they're finding that the health effects of food are likely derived from the synergistic interactions of nutrients and other compounds within and among the foods we eat. This has led to a shift from nutrient based recommendations toward guidelines based on foods and eating patterns. There's no single healthy diet. Many eating patterns sustain good health. What they have in common is lots of fruits, vegetables and whole grains, along with healthy sources of protein and fats. Consistently eating foods like these will help lower your risk for conditions such as heart disease, stroke, diabetes and certain forms of cancer.

If you'd like to make this largely plant based approach to eating one of your good health goals, well, here's how to get started. First, build a better plate. The healthy eating plate is made up of one half vegetables and fruits, one quarter whole grains and one quarter healthy protein. Whole and healthy are important words here. Refined grains think white breads, pastas and rice have less fiber and fewer nutrients than whole grains such as whole wheat, bread and brown rice. Healthy proteins include fish, poultry, beans and nuts, but not red meats or processed meats. Many studies have shown that red meat and especially processed meats are linked with colorectal cancer and that you can lower your risk for heart disease by replacing either type of meat with healthier protein sources.

So eat red meat sparingly, selecting the leanest cuts and avoid processed meats altogether. Secondly, pile on the vegetables and fruits. Vegetables and fruits are high in fiber and contain many vitamins and minerals, as well as hundreds of beneficial plant chemicals or phytochemicals that you can't get in supplements. Diets rich in vegetables and fruit can benefit the heart by lowering blood pressure, cholesterol levels and inflammation and improving insulin resistance and blood vessel function. In long term observational studies, people who eat more fruits and vegetables have a lower risk of heart disease, diabetes and weight gain. And those who eat more fruit also have a lower risk of stroke.

Thirdly, go for the good fat. At one time we were told to eat less fat, but now we know that it's mainly the type of fat that counts. The most beneficial sources are plants and fish. You can help lower bad LDL cholesterol by eating mostly polyunsaturated fats, including vegetable oils and omega three fatty acids found in fish seeds and nuts and canola oil and monounsaturated fats and avocados and many plant based oils such as olive oil and canola oil. Saturated fats mostly found in dairy and meat products and trans fats, hydrogenated fat found in many fried and baked goods boost LDL cholesterol and triglycerides, increasing your risk of heart disease. We're still trans fats.

Reduce your good HDL cholesterol. Next, drink enough water. Many foods contain water, so you may get enough every day without making a special effort. But it can be helpful to drink water or something else. No calorie liquid such as black tea, coffee or carbonated water with meals or as an alternative to snacking. A reasonable goal is four to six cups of water a day. Finally, eat breakfast. It's easy to skip breakfast when you're in a rush, aren't hungry or want to cut calories. But a healthy morning meal makes for smaller rises in blood sugar and insulin throughout the day, which can lower your risk of overeating and impulse snacking. Eating breakfast every day is one characteristic common to participants in the National Weight Control Registry, who have lost at least 30 pounds and kept the weight off longer than a year.

So should you take supplements? In the 1980s, many nutritionists and some physicians began to recommend and take vitamin supplements. However, as described in a cast of characters Vitamin E to zinc, the evidence for the health benefits of most supplements is not strong. Notable exceptions are fish oil for cardiovascular disease and vitamin D for bone health. Although foods that contain vitamin A and beta carotene as well as vitamins B, C and E are clearly good for health. Taking supplements of these vitamins has no proven health benefits. What about a simple multivitamin? These pills, which also usually contain multiple minerals, are the most popular among all dietary supplements.

50 percent of Americans take them on a regular basis, shelling out more than 20 billion dollars annually on these products. On an individual basis, a daily multivitamin won't set you back that much. A year's supply of many popular brands costs about thirty dollars. However, despite widespread belief that it is multivitamin. Will prevent chronic diseases such as cancer and heart disease. There's no evidence to support such claims. The National Institutes of Health convened a meeting on multivitamin and mineral supplements in May 2006. The state of the science statement and issued was extremely cautious.

Present evidence is insufficient to recommend either for or against the use of multivitamins, multi mineral supplements by the American public to prevent chronic disease. The experts noted that the heaviest users of vitamins and minerals supplements are Americans who probably need them the least. Those who are well-educated have higher incomes, exercise and already have healthy diets. A 2008 study in the Archives of Internal Medicine tracked nearly one hundred and sixty two thousand participants in the Women's Health Initiative and found that multivitamins have no effect whatsoever in 10 health related categories, including cancer, heart attack and stroke.

Supplement makers didn't live any longer either. Here are some potential dangers of consuming supplements. Number one, potential pitfalls. Number two, more isn't always better. Now let's talk about potential pitfalls. Shopping for any kind of supplement can be confusing. A staggering array of multivitamins and other supplements crowd the shelves of pharmacies, grocery stores and specialty stores, and many more are now available over the Internet before you buy. It's wise to realize that some of these products may offer much more or possibly less than you really need to enhance your health. Dietary supplements may legally contain vitamins, minerals, herbs, amino acids, enzymes, organ tissues and a few other substances.

In short, practically any ingredient is promoted as a way to bolster your diet and presumably your health. The FDA does not certify supplements for safety or effectiveness the way it monitors drugs under the Dietary Supplement Health and Education Act of 1994. The FDA cannot approve supplements or demand that manufacturers undertake rigorous studies to prove their worth. The FDA doesn't set potency or dosage standards either. Manufacturers are left to police themselves and before a worrisome supplement can be pulled off the market. The FDA has to prove that it creates a significant health risk. This can be a problem, as is made clear by a January 2009 consumer lab report.

The consumer watchdog organization tested the quality and contents of 29 of the leading multivitamin and multi mineral products for adults and children sold in the United States and Canada. Eight products did not meet. The claims stated on their labels had other quality issues, while another 12 provided levels that may be too high for healthy people. For example, one man's multivitamin supplement contained just over 2000 micrograms of folic acid, which is twice the safe upper limit for that vitamin. While supplement manufacturers can't legally claim to prevent, treat or cure specific diseases, they can come pretty close.

They're allowed to make structure function claims that sound impressive to most consumers. A product may build strong teeth or improve memory or boost the immune system. Manufacturers can make these assertions without supplying a stitch of proof to any agency. Your cue for healthy skepticism should be the words printed alongside. This statement has not been evaluated by the Food and Drug Administration. Certain health claims, backed by substantial scientific agreement and not limited to particular brands, can appear on supplement bottles. For example, supplement manufacturers can advertise that calcium helps protect against osteoporosis and folic acid may prevent neural tube defects in fetuses.

Because these statements are borne out by science and have been carefully evaluated. Also, more isn't always better. Many people who take supplements subscribe to the idea that more is better without carefully considering the arguments for or against their choices. They may take a handful of other supplements along with their multivitamin. At best, they may be wasting their money. At worst, they may be endangering their health. Take vitamin C and A, for example, once your blood level of vitamin C reaches the saturation point which occurs, if you take about 200 milligrams per day, your body usually excretes the excess. That's why vitamin C toxicity rarely occurs. However, people who consistently take too much vitamin A won't be as fortunate because fat soluble vitamins remain in the body they can more easily build to toxic levels.

A pregnant woman who takes too much vitamin A risks birth defects to her fetus excess. Vitamin A also compromises bone health and blood clotting, and it can overstimulate your immune system. Many consumers are spurred to take excessive doses by overenthusiastic news stories on the potential benefits of certain vitamins and minerals. Remember, though, that the good news from the latest study may eventually prove true, or it may be refuted by other studies, often promising test tube and animal studies don't pan out in people, and certain types of human studies offer more definitive information than others.

Sometimes exciting results from initial observational studies aren't confirmed by randomized controlled trials, which are considered the gold standard of research. And even these studies often have their limitations. It's generally safest to wait for evidence to accumulate before jumping on the supplements. Bandwagon. Consider the potential risks, possible benefits and costs. What about specialized supplements aimed at women, men and seniors? While some of these supplements may be helpful in certain cases, others are merely marketing gimmicks designed to enhance profits rather than your health products vary wildly.

Read the labels to make sure you get what you need while staying within safe limits. If you're a woman, which vitamins and minerals are most helpful for you? Well, that depends partly on your age and on childbearing concerns. Folic acid supplements are necessary if there's a chance that you could become pregnant and iron is important for you if you're still menstruating. It's essential that you get enough folic acid to prevent birth defects called neural tube defects, which develop in the earliest days and weeks of pregnancy because not every pregnancy is planned. Most experts suggest that all women capable of becoming pregnant take a daily multivitamin that has at least 400 micrograms of folic acid.

Your doctor may suggest taking more than that amount if you plan to get pregnant and have previously had a child with a neural tube defect to replace iron lost during monthly periods, you need a multivitamin or women's supplement with iron. Iron deficiency saps your energy, eventually leaving you weak and tired. In the United States, one in 10 women and girls who menstruate are deficient in iron. The recommended daily amount of iron for adult women ages 19 to 50 is 18 milligrams. If you're pregnant, you need larger amounts of certain vitamins and minerals, particularly iron and folic acid, prenatal vitamins, which can be purchased by prescription or over the counter.

Meet these needs. It is important not to take other supplements unless specifically advised by a qualified healthcare professional. The earliest weeks of pregnancy are crucial in the fetus's development. So the sooner and during pregnancy you start taking a prenatal vitamin, the better. If you plan to get pregnant or learn that you are, talk with your doctor right away to find out which prenatal supplement would be best for you to take during pregnancy. Your iron requirements increased to 27 milligrams and your folic acid requirement to 600 micrograms. The calcium RDA remains at 1000 milligrams for women ages 19 and over, although some clinicians suggest adding calcium during pregnancy for extra insurance.

As for women who reached menopause, unless your doctor advises otherwise, you can switch to a supplement that reduces or eliminates iron. Diet alone should supply enough iron and prevent a possible iron overload. Iron overload can damage the liver and other body tissues, causing diabetes, heart disease, arthritis and liver cancer. More likely, supplements designed for older women typically have little or no iron and more calcium and vitamin D. After menopause or hysterectomy, you need only eight milligrams of iron daily, many extra shy away from any iron supplementation for men. That's because men like women who no longer menstruate aren't typically losing much iron.

For that reason, supplements aimed specifically at men generally reduce iron or drop it from the formula. This can help prevent iron overload, which can stem from taking more iron than necessary through supplements. Iron overload may also occur because of a common genetic defect that occurs more often in men than women. Iron overload can damage the liver and other body tissues, raising the risk for diabetes, heart disease, arthritis and liver cancer. Men's multivitamin and mineral formulations typically add or increase selenium and lycopene, too, which may protect against prostate cancer and other types of cancer.

Some drop calcium entirely. Formulas with low or no calcium are fine for men as long as they get adequate amounts of calcium in their diets to prevent osteoporosis. Exercise coupled with vitamin D and vitamin K is more important for bone health in men, products aimed at older people tend to boost the amount of certain B vitamins, partly because many elderly men and women have trouble absorbing vitamin B 12. These products also tend to add antioxidants and often vitamin D and selenium. There's little evidence to support the value of antioxidant supplements. Some experts recommend getting at least 2000 IU of vitamin D daily after age 70. As you age, your skin loses some of its ability to produce vitamin D from sunlight, and many older people don't spend that much time in the sun.

As for selenium, evidence suggests no benefit to this mineral until more information is available or unless your doctor gives you other advice. A daily multivitamin should offer enough B vitamins. However, if you're over 70 and get little sun exposure, you may need to add a separate vitamin D supplement. Detoxification is a normal process within the body as it neutralizes and eliminates toxins through the major organs such as our colon, liver, kidney, lungs, lymph and skin. Our bodies do it naturally every day. In fact, it's one of our most basic automatic functions.

But what if our self-cleaning systems are overloaded by our unhealthy lifestyle and exposure to environmental toxins? According to many healing experts, detoxification through special cleansing programs may be the missing link to disease prevention, especially for immune deficiency diseases like cancer, arthritis, diabetes, chronic fatigue syndrome and Candida. Our chemical diet has an overabundance of animal protein too. Much saturated fat and too much caffeine and alcohol radically alters our internal ecosystem, but even if your diet is good, a cleanse can restore your immune system and protect yourself against environmental toxins that pave the way for disease-bearing bacteria, viruses and parasites in the animal kingdom and in traditional cultures.

Routine fasting and allowing the body time to clean itself out has been a normal practice. Just think how many showers you take a year to clean the outside of your body and then how many cleanses you do in a year to clean the inside of your body. Here's a quick detox plan for you on rising. Take a large glass and have the juice out of one fresh lemon and crush a thumbnail size of fresh ginger. Fill the rest of the glass with room temperature or warm water before starting work and breakfast mix wheatgrass or barley, grass, powder and spring water to make a green drink to alkalize and energize the cells of your body and accelerate the cleansing process.

It'll taste a little weird to start with, but as your bloodstream levels drop, your taste buds will adjust to the flavor for breakfast. Break your fast with a fresh vegetable juice of four medium sized carrots, one beetroot, one cucumber, one handful of baby spinach and one quarter cup parsley. Take one thousand milligrams of vitamin C and 1000 mg. Flaxseed oil capsules between breakfast and lunch have a caffeine free detox, tea of peppermint, ginseng, licorice, root, ginger or camomile or a special natural laxative tea, more green drink as you need it during lunch.

Have a small to medium serving of brown rice with a mixture of raw and steamed vegetables, choose from broccoli, shiitake mushrooms, bok choy, radishes, rocket spring onions, watercress, garlic and ginger, seasoned with sea greens and flavor with one cup of miso soup or lemon juice and extra virgin olive oil. Take one 1000 mg tablet of vitamin C in mid-afternoon. Have another vegetable juice of carrot, apple and ginger to boost your energy levels for early dinner. Have a freshly squeezed vegetable juice of two carrots, two tomatoes, a handful of spinach leaves, two celery ribs, half a cucumber and half a green bell pepper. Add one tablespoon of wheat grass or barley powder. Take one 1000 milligram tablet of vitamin C before bed.

Relax your body with a detox, tea of peppermint, ginseng, licorice, root, ginger or camomile tea or freshman and green tea with cardamom pods. And there you have it. Follow this program as closely as possible for a minimum of three days to really see the results. You can experiment with the vegetable juices throughout the day, but just make sure you're not adding too many sweet fruits. Ideally, none at all, as these add to the sugar or acidic load in the body, which is what we're trying to avoid during this cleanse. So what's the recipe? One detox meal consists of pesto, mushroom and black olive top. A nod to detox water consists of slimmed down detox, water and watermelon detox water.

Here's the recipe for pesto mushroom, 20 button mushrooms or four portobello mushrooms. One cup walnuts, one half cup pine nuts, three cups basil, one half cup olive oil, two to three cloves of garlic, one teaspoon of sea salt and two tablespoons of lemon juice substitutes. You can use a rocket to fill out the basil if you're short. And here's the cooking method: one wash and stem the mushrooms and lay out on a serving plate to place all remaining ingredients in a food processor and blend until Smooth three, fill the mushrooms with pesto and serve fresh for if desired for a more crispy taste dehydrate for five to six hours. Mushrooms are one of the best natural sources of niacin, which is essential for energy production, brain function and the skin.

It also helps in balancing blood sugar levels and lowering cholesterol. Nuts, seeds and their cold pressed oils should be included in your diet on a regular basis as they contain high levels of the essential fatty acids or eephus or good fats. Additionally, they're also a powerhouse of nutrients and contain high forms of digestible protein antioxidant vitamins ABC and E calcium, magnesium, potassium, zinc, iron, selenium and manganese. So what about black olive tapenade? Simple three cups of , black olives, one half cup olive oil, one small handful parsley optional, two tablespoons of lemon juice, three cloves, garlic and one tablespoon sea salt. Firstly, one process everything except olives in a blender or food processor until smooth to add olives and pulse until olives are roughly chopped.

Three to serve as a dip with flax crackers, olives and olive oil are very rich in antioxidants. Antioxidants deactivate free radicals, allowing us to live longer, overcome illness and maintain more acute mental and muscular faculties. Olive's display antifungal and antibacterial properties and are used in a detoxifying diet. Garlic contains high doses of natural sulfur or. MSM MSM provides elasticity, movement, healing and repair within the tissues, it greatly enhances the structural integrity of connective tissue and joint cartilage and has been shown to reverse arthritic conditions, including pain and inflammation. MSM is renowned as a beautifying nutrient, the best natural food cosmetic in the world.

MSM, through its ability to continuously build and rebuild perfect collagen and keratin, is able to make our hair, nails and skin shine with radiance. You can buy MSM on its own, which we recommend as a supplement to a healthy diet. The powder tastes awful, so we'd suggest the capsule's parsley is a nutrient powerhouse containing more vitamin C than citrus fruit. It even contains vitamin B 12, mostly thought to be only bioavailable in dairy and meat products. B 12, apart from being found in parsley, is also available in blue. Green algae inspire Alina, and it's normally synthesized in the intestine. When in abundance and healthy bacteria is present, BE2 is needed in the body from making use of protein and helps the blood carry oxygen.

Also, here's the recipe for slimmed down detox water. One half gallon springwater, one half grapefruit sliced in half cucumber sliced two to three mint leaves, one half lemon sliced and one half lime sliced. Simply combine all the ingredients in a pitcher. Allow the ingredients to chill in the refrigerator for one to two hours before serving drinks throughout the day or discard after twenty four hours. Here's what you need for watermelon, detox, water, two cups, seedless watermelon cubes and four cups of water. Firstly place the watermelon in a pitcher and cover with water. Let it sit for a few hours in the refrigerator before drinking so the water gets all the nice watermelon flavor.

Lastly, here's the recipe for raspberry and mint scented water to liters. Cold spring water or filtered tap water, two tablespoons, raspberries, fresh or frozen, two tablespoons, fresh mint leaves and one lime to get more flavor and juice out of your lime. Microwaved for thirty seconds. One cool slice, please. Raspberries, mint, lime and water in a large jug stir and serve. And there you have it. All the knowledge you need on supplements and a secret detox plan and recipes.

How To Get Rid Of Love Handles

In this chapter, you'll learn how to get rid of love handles, so what are the workouts for women? Firstly, crunches on an exercise ball. What are the steps? Sit on a well inflated exercise ball. For more information on what diameter ball to use, read ball size matters. Place your hands behind your head and walk your feet away from the ball so your torso starts to roll onto the ball. The ball should support your hips and the curve of your lower back. Your legs should form a bridge with your knees bent at right angles. Exhale and lift your upper body by about 45 degrees, pulling the deep abs in toward the spine and return to the starting position. Don't yank your neck and do twenty five reps.

The second exercise is to palletize one by lying on your back with your legs in tabletop position, hips and knees at right angles. Engage your deep abs to round your lower spine into the floor. Make sure you're not pushing your abs, which means you're just working the top layer of abs, which is a palletize no no. Exhale and lift your upper back off the floor until the bottom tips of your shoulder blades. Skim the floor, straighten your legs to a 45 degree angle, but make sure your low back is staying connected to the floor. Reach your arms towards your feet. Your arms will be about two inches off the floor. Pump your arms up and down with a small range of motion, keeping your elbows straight, inhale for five arm pumps and exhale for five arm pumps. That completes one set or cycle.

Repeat the cycle nine more times for a total of one hundred pumps. Keep your upper body stable while your arms pump. The third exercise is bicycle crunches lie flat on the floor with your lower back pressed to the ground. Pull your abs down to also target your deep abs, interlace your fingers and put your hands behind your head. Bring your knees in towards your chest and lift your shoulder blades off the ground. Straighten your right leg out to about a 45 degree angle to the ground while turning your upper body to the left, bringing your right elbow toward the left knee. Make sure your ribcage is moving and not just your elbows.

Now switch sides and do the same motion on the other side to complete one rep and to create the pedaling motion. Do this exercise with slow and controlled motion. Do ten to twenty reps. The fourth exercise is twisting side planks, come into a side plank on your right side with your feet stacked one on top of the other and your weight on your right elbow with your fingers reaching away from your body. Palm down, place your left arm behind your head and inhale to prepare, exhale and pull your navel to your spine to engage your deep abs and rotate your left rib cage toward the floor. Stay there for a second and deepen your abdominal connection by pulling your navel in towards your spine even more, return to the starting position and repeat seven more times for a total of eight reps.

Then switch sides and repeat the series again on both sides. The fifth exercise is the Russian twist. Sit on the ground with your knees bent and your heels about a foot from your bum. Lean slightly back without rounding your spine at all. It is really important and difficult to keep your back straight, but don't let it curve. Place your arms straight out in front of you with your hands. One on top of the other. Your hands should be level with the bottom of your ribcage, pull your navel to your spine and twist slowly to the left. The movement is not large and comes from the ribs rotating, not from your arms swinging. Inhale through the center and rotate to the right. This completes one rep. Do 16 full rotations to get washboard abs.

The best exercise is hanging AB curls using a pull up bar. Get a good grip with your palms facing outward toward each other. Start with your legs hanging straight down and on and exhale. Pull your abs toward your spine and bend your knees, lifting them towards your chest without swinging slowly. Lower your knees. Returning to a straight leg position, repeat for a total of ten to twelve reps. Next, we'll talk about the best exercises for men. The first is, Of course, sit ups lie flat on your back, on the floor, with your knees bent and your legs secured under a piece of heavy furniture. I'm assuming that you're doing this routine at home. Place your hands by your chest, flexing your abdominals, raise your torso until you are nearly in a sitting position, retaining tension on the abs, lower your torso to the beginning position.

Remember to maintain full control throughout the movement. Also avoid the temptation to rock back and forth. The second exercise is leg raises. Lie flat on your back, on the floor, with your legs straight out in front of you. Place your hands at your sides by the floor for support, flexing your lower abdominals, raise your legs until they're perpendicular to the floor, retaining tension on the abs, lower your legs to the beginning position again. Maintain full control throughout the movement. Avoid the temptation to let your legs drop on the negative portion of the movement. The third exercise is knees in, sit on the floor or on the edge of a chair or.

Sized bench with your legs extended in front of you and your hands holding onto the sides for support, keeping your knees together, pull your knees in towards your chest until you can go no further, keeping the tension on your lower AB muscles returned to the start position and repeat the movement until you have completed your set. The fourth exercise is Tolj touchers. Sit on the floor or on the edge of a chair or exercise bench with your legs extended in front of you and your hands holding onto the sides for support simultaneously. Bring your legs up as far as possible, while at the same time bringing your torso towards them. Return to the start position and repeat the movement until you have completed your set note. This is a modified version of a V up in a true V up.

Your starting position is lying down on the floor and bringing yourself up with no arms support. The fifth exercise is crunches lie flat on your back, on the floor with your legs in front of you bent at the knees, placed your hands by your chest. At this time, raise your shoulders and torso as far as possible from the ground in a curling movement without raising your back from the floor, retaining tensions on the abs. Bring your torso to the starting position. To slim down, you have to alter your energy balance. There are simply two ways to accomplish this. Either take in less calories or spend more energy through exercise. The easiest way to boil down your consumption is merely to cut back on the size of your meals and or the total high calorie foods you eat.

This doesn't mean that you have to give up any certain food. Bear in mind that there's more to a beautiful body than just utilizing effective wellness products. You need to be on a total preventative health care and wellness program that involves diet, nutrition, making a point that your body gets the proper nutrients and exercise. Optimum body functions today require any added help they can get as most people don't go through the trouble to consume foods that are healthy and beneficial for them. Therefore, there's a need to make a conscious effort to sort out essential vitamin types of foods and include them into the daily diet plan for good conditions.

Everyone Wants Success

Everyone wants success, but is it for everyone? Experts will tell you that anyone can be successful at anything they want only if they put their mind to it. But is that how success works? Is it really that simple? Not exactly. If anything, success comes at a cost. Most people never become successful because they're not willing to pay the price of success. It's a choice they have to make when they have to step out of the box, make some changes to their existing lifestyle, drop old habits and pick up new ones and invest effort, attitude and morale to keep things going. But if you're willing to learn and transform yourself in all the right areas, then success is definitely for you. So to find out how you can do that, let's get started.

Set BIG Goals

In this chapter, we'll talk about setting big goals. If you're going to set yourself up for success in life, then you need to set some mighty meaningful goals for yourself. So as a starting point, the first and foremost thing to remember on the journey of personal success is a positive attitude towards everything. If you fail once, brush up your knees and get back out there. If you get rejected the first time, better yourself with a positive outlook. Prove yourself, instead of bringing yourself down with negativity, tell yourself through every obstacle and hardship. I did not come this far to only come this far now success is achieved overnight. No mountain is climbed without a few falls or two.

If others can put up a fight to achieve personal success despite countless hardships. So can you better aim high and miss than to aim low and achieve? It's always better to aim high, even if you don't succeed at first. When you aim big, you dream big and tell yourself that you stand a chance against all odds. The problem with setting lower standards is that the lower you set your aim, the more you can find yourself. You miss more chances and more of your abilities are left unknown. Likewise, more of your will goes without a test where you could achieve the stars.

Your low aim of never going that high will hold you back. No matter how many people look down on you and doubt your capability, it's your own personal belief, unwavering resilience and ambitions that lead you to achieving your ultimate dream.

But the moment you start to doubt yourself, the moment you decide you can't aim higher for the fear of failure is when your downfall begins with a higher aim. You may miss it first, or you may make it on your first try. Take your chances of leap of faith in yourself. The higher you aim, the more you achieve. Even if you fall short of your goal, you won't end up too far from it. Just think of achieving a good score on a test. If you aim low at getting a fifty percent mark on your test, you might be successful and achieve that. But that's all it will be.

An average and low achievement. If you aim higher at getting ninety percent, you may miss and hit eighty, which is still higher and so much better than the low set aim of fifty percent. The same goes for all tests and trials. Life puts you through set purpose driven goals. When setting goals, you need to think about how to achieve them, what you need to do to achieve them, and how much time you need to get there. But the real driving force that will actually make you sweat for any goal is why you need to achieve that goal. Why is it a priority? Why is it so important? Setting goals is easy. Just think of drawing up a New Year's resolution. Everyone does that every year and has been doing it forever, so much so that it's become a mere habit and nothing much else.

But what people don't do is pause to think over the goal and question why, inevitably, without this driving force, they'll soon forget all about it. As such, it's important to not merely set goals but set purpose driven goals. Instead, for example, you may well be thinking of hitting the gym, working out and getting yourself in shape with just this in mind. You set a goal in your New Year's resolution to workout every day. So you do it the first day and the second, and then something comes up on the third. Then you end up skipping the fourth day because you get lazy and there goes your fitness. There goes the goal.

On the other hand, an obese person on the verge of getting diabetes and a possible heart attack is told by a doctor he needs to work out to lose weight really soon if he still wants a chance at a healthy life or maybe just life. This is his why? This is why he won't skip the third or fourth day no matter what comes up. This is why he will achieve his goal with more determination. So through every hardship on your way, when you are at the brink of giving up, you can tell yourself again and again why you cannot give up, why you must go on, give yourself a time frame to work with without setting a time frame to achieve any particular goal. There will be no sense of urgency.

The importance of getting anything done is great, but the importance of getting it done in time is even greater. Giving yourself a duration for a specific task will make you more productive in that short time, then you would be without it. If you know the deadline for a task is twenty four hours, you'll make yourself attend to that task as a priority. You'll utilize those twenty four hours in the most effective way possible to complete the task on hand. If you set a deadline of one week for the. The same task, not only will you waste the entire week and be less productive, you will also waste precious time that you could have used to complete other tasks as well. Having said that, the time frame has to be realistic and attainable. You need to be sure whether the goal is a short term goal or a long term one.

Losing 10 kilograms in three days. Not possible. Not attainable. Even if you spend most of the hours of the three days in the gym, the time frame should not be based on some delusion and understanding of the goal. The priority you're willing to give it can help you decide better how much time you need to give it and how much time is sensible to give it. If you have an essay due next week and you keep delaying it or doing it in bits paragraph to paragraph a day, it'll get tiresome and boring. In the end, it might not even make a lot of sense. Plus, you'll lose the sense of urgency that would make you more productive. But if you decide to do it in two days, you'll utilize those two days much more effectively and we'll even have time for other goals. Once you finish with that essay, the less you linger on with the task at hand, the better.

Make Real Decisions

In this chapter, we'll discuss making real decisions. Everyone has to make decisions in their daily life, while some of them are small. Others are big and have a profound impact on your life. So it's very important to evaluate all aspects of an issue before coming to a decision. There are a few things that, if considered, can help you make good decisions that you won't regret later in life. Make smart decisions. Most people don't realize the importance little decisions have in life. When you make a decision, it initiates events in your life that unfold into either something good or bad. Depending on whether your decision was smart or not, you must make smart decisions. It often happens that we make decisions based on what others think or how a certain thing is supposed to be.

The people around you have a huge impact on your decision making skills. Surround yourself with a positive presence. There's no right way to make a smart decision. The process of making a smart decision varies from person to person. For some people, their gut plays a role in making the best decision. The first thought that they have is the best for them. If they overthink the issue, they end up blowing the problem out of proportion and making decisions that are unnecessary. But for others, thinking is an important part of decision making. They need to think about a problem and make sure they've got everything covered before they decide something.

Whichever of the two you are, make sure you cover every aspect of the decision. If you make smart decisions, your life will be much better and easier. Most people suffer the consequences of decisions made poorly or in haste. Take your time and get to know the issues in depth. Once you are content with your decision, proceed to its application. Just don't rush into making a decision. If you decide to move into a new house, make sure you ask yourself whether it helps you. Will you be paying more rent? Is this house close to your workplace? Is it too big or small for you? When you make a smart decision, you have no regrets. Later, think everything through when you decide to move into this place.

Otherwise, you're faced with problems like transportation issues, extra expenditure on rent and waste or lack of space. Carry out your decisions. People are always making decisions about the changes they want to bring in life, but often end up ignoring them. You must carry out your decision. If you have strong willpower and you're dedicated to something, you'll surely be able to carry it out. For example, if you decide to join a book club in your local library, push yourself to do it as soon as possible. When you delay something, the chances of it never happening increase. Go to the library the first chance you get and fill out the membership form. A very common example in this regard is of smokers.

There are so many people out there who want to quit smoking. They've searched everything and they've planned everything out, but they fail to carry out their decision. If you keep postponing it, you'll never be able to achieve it. Why start tomorrow when you can do it? Today, you can quit smoking if you put your heart and mind into it, just go cold turkey. There are so many others who have done it. Read the stories of people online or join a help group so that you have the motivation you need. Interacting with people who have succeeded in carrying out their decisions will help you immensely. Don't give up if you fail the first time. Learn from the mistakes you make in the first attempt.

Ask yourself how can you succeed next time? Remember that you can do it. Nothing or no one can stop you. If you put your mind to something, keep reminding yourself that this is a smart decision that you made and now you need to act on it. It's the first step that counts the most every day. You might tell yourself that you'll start tomorrow once you decide that you're going to do it. Today is when you succeed. Just take that first step and the road will lead on. Don't look back. It's not always easy to carry out your decisions. Sometimes you even start. But there are hurdles in the way. If you want to quit smoking, you might be peer pressured to derail from this decision or people around.

You could tell you that one smoker day doesn't do any harm. You need to remember why you started in the first place before you made this decision. You must have thought a lot about the health and social changes it will bring in your life every time you feel like you are derailing from your path. Remember why you started the journey in the first place. You might even have to cut off things and people in order to carry out your decisions, cut out people from your life who pressure you into smoking. It might be hard at first, but you need to remember that these people are toxic for you.

If someone's bringing negativity in your life, why keep them close? Why did you decide to volunteer at a shelter? Because it made you content and you wanted to spend your time doing something good. Don't let laziness or a lack of a proper schedule. Derail you from this decision, don't let your laziness stop you from doing things that are good for you, sometimes you make mistakes when you carry out a decision. Don't let that stop you from continuing. Make amends and carry on. So start making smart decisions and carry them out without stopping for anyone or anything.

Consistency Is Key

In this chapter, we'll discuss how consistency is key. Consistency is the magic ingredient for success, be it personal betterment, business academics or just the relationships with loved ones without consistency and the will to stay steadfast in what you're trying to achieve. There is no success. A child never learns to tie his shoelaces the very first try. He tries over and over again until he finally figures it out on the hundredth time. The important thing is not to do it once, but to do it over and over again, to never stop till you reach your goal, be committed and persevere.

Perseverance is to keep up your efforts and doing something, no matter the difficulties and obstacles in the way it is. Perseverance that helps you learn how to walk, then helps you study for an exam or makes you get up every single day and get on with your life. Just like solving a jigsaw puzzle. If the piece doesn't fit, try another one and then another one until it's completed. Similarly, all goals are left unachieved, all success unknown till one learns to stay committed and persevere. Push yourself to be patient and stay committed.

Tell yourself why it's important that you stay steadfast. Remind yourself of why you must go on. Anyone can try once and give up, but only those who stay committed and persevere succeed in life in being persistent towards achieving any goal in life. You learn from your failures. You learn what went wrong the first time. You learn how to defeat these obstacles rather than be defeated by them. Everything in life demands this commitment from a successful career to a healthy relationship. Without it, a medical student would give up the first time they failed to memorize the horrid details of a gruesome disease.

Without it, a mother would wake up every single night to nurse her child the moment he or she lets out a cry. And to be honest, without it, wedding vows wouldn't mean much either. Have a routine for success. Having a routine is vital for success in general, without proper division and allotment of time you give to a particular task every day, there's no way of achieving consistency. It should be such that your mind automatically rings a bell to remind you what you must be doing at that particular hour. For instance, think of your daily skin regimen before bed. To have a routine would mean having dinner on time, cleaning up the kitchen next, and then heading to the bedroom to follow up with your skincare routine.

Without a routine. A change in the timing of one thing would lead to a change in the other. With a late dinner, you might end up too exhausted and miss out on your daily routine. We all know how that goes. Then it's missing out one day, then the next and so on. So everything does need a proper allocation of time. What time do you wake up? How long do you work out for what time do you eat? How much time can you afford to give to your hobbies? Are you giving enough time to friends and family? All of this needs to be set in order to achieve success. Being consistent with the routine maximizes the benefits of all the hard work. In the long term.

Having a messed up routine will not only stand in your way of success, but also mess up other aspects of life as well. Create good habits. Being consistent leads to the development of good habits. Creating good habits ensures success in all areas of life. Doing something once in a while or when you get the time doesn't get you anywhere near achieving your aims and aspirations. Instead, the keys to achieving any goals you set for our consistency and making quick decisions. This decision to do something every day is, in other words, your habits. The first thing to keep in mind for creating good habits is to choose discipline and your priority over your moods. I'm not in the mood to study today.

Might as well binge watch a series. I'm a bit upset about working out today. Skipping one day shouldn't hurt. We've all been there. We've all chosen the mood over consistency, which has eventually led to a failure in developing good habits to help keep the good habits you create. It's a good idea to track your progress. This helps you know how beneficial the habit has been for you. The clearer you see the results, the stronger you will be to continue them. For example, if you have a goal set on your weight and how much you want to lose, keeping a record every week should help you see a clear pattern of the good that is coming from your habit of exercise.

When you see the actual figure on scale, you'll get more enthusiastic and positive about your workout and how it turns out for, you know, results can be seen overnight. Nothing is achieved in one go. Achievements take long persistence, struggle. Success isn't out of reach. It's only difficult to reach through persistence, perseverance and commitment. Success can be guaranteed. Consistency leads to the development of good habits. Good habits lead to action. And that gets all the work done once you get used to the struggle and of staying steadfast, no matter the difficulties, no failures can set you back. They only make you stronger and more ambitious than ever to reach your goals.

How To Be Accountable

In this chapter, we'll learn how to be accountable. There comes a certain time of your life when you realize that now you are accountable for everything you do. The idea is quite daunting as accountability is needed in all spheres of life. In some situations, you have to be accountable for yourself alone, while in others you're accountable for others as well. Take responsibility. The first step of being accountable is to take responsibility. Now, it might be a personal responsibility or one that affects others around you. For instance, if you're the head of a family, you have to be accountable to them or if you're leading an excursion tour, you have to be accountable to your tour group.

Remember this with great power comes great responsibility. So take full responsibility for your actions and don't make excuses. If something goes wrong, you need to realize that you're in charge and it's only you who's accountable. So take the responsibility of your actions and theirs too. It's easy to throw someone else under the bus for anything that goes wrong, but the mature thing to do is to take responsibility rather than make excuses. The tour didn't reach its destination on time. Are you going to blame someone from the group for not coming on time, or are you going to take responsibility for not making the instructions clear enough? The choice is up to you. Always remember it is mature to be accountable for yourself.

It might not be the best feeling in the world at the time being, but you will feel much content later. Say it out loud that you'll do it. Positive affirmation is very important, so it's crucial to keep reminding yourself that you will do it. Sometimes you get sidetracked by events or people, but you mustn't let this be permanent. You're also accountable to yourself for your mission or goal in life. You have to determine what you want to do or achieve in life. Ask yourself what you're good at or what you like. Base your goals and long term plans on your capabilities, desires and strengths. Make a mission statement for yourself. Write it down somewhere so that you can read it every day.

Many people have inspirational quotes on their walls or phone screen so that they look at them every day. And this way they get inspired everyday, even on ones that are not so good. But if you're someone with a knack for writing, write down your goals. Make sure to write it in a place where you can see it every day. If it stares you in the face, you can't run away from it. Or if you have supportive peers, get feedback from them. Ask them if you're doing things right or if you need to improve. This will help remind you that you need to do better. Also, it will give you an insight into how others perceive your efforts. If you're in a workplace, your subordinates can also tell you how well you're doing. If the feedback is positive, it'll motivate you to do even better and have a sense of accomplishment.

And if the feedback is not positive, you can use it to improve performance as you're the one who will eventually be accountable. Either way, feedback can do wonders if only to hold yourself accountable. Be honest, just as accountability is important, so is honesty. It's very important to be honest about the results. When you're working alone or in a team, you have to stay honest about the outcome of your efforts. Success only becomes possible when you own up to your mistakes. While they can be cumbersome, mistakes are also valuable learning opportunities.

If you've done something wrong, ask yourself why it happened and what you can do to make it right. If you totally ignore it or lie about it to yourself and others, how can you ever hope to rectify it? Plus, when you're not honest with yourself, you'll always have a constant feeling of dissatisfaction. Your conscience won't let you forget it. So wouldn't it be better to just admit it? Also, be honest about the goals you set. Be realistic. Holding yourself accountable for your actions is also a reality check to set goals that are attainable. Realism is essential when setting goals. So you want to save money for a car and you tell yourself that you will do it in a year's time.

Now you need to be real about it. Do you have enough income coming in every month that you can save some of it for buying a car? Are you ready to cut out some expenses so that you can save? Will you be able to manage it in a year or do you need more time? If you think your goals are realistic, proceed with them. Then if you fail to buy a car in twelve months, don't make excuses or blame something else for it. Ask yourself why you weren't able to do it. Maybe you set the wrong time frame or misspent the money that you could have saved on unnecessary things.

Be fully honest with yourself about the results of your personal quest or team work. A good way to prevent disappointment or unpleasant situations is to have a plan B, so. You could fix things later, being accountable can be a frightening thought because no one likes to be judged, especially for something that someone else did. But if you follow the right strategy and put in the effort, you'll be able to master the art of accountability.

Nothing Is Impossible

In this chapter, we'll talk about how nothing is impossible. Everyone says that nothing is impossible, but do they actually believe it? If you really want everything to be possible, you have to start believing it. You'd be surprised by the power that belief has in life. You can make everything possible if you condition your mind to think so, condition your mind to think. Positive optimism is an essential part of success in life. Once you condition your mind to think well and good, it'll have a positive impact on all your decisions and thoughts. You might look at someone making art and think to yourself that it's possible for you to do that. Why do you have to think so? A better way to go about it is to tell yourself that you can do just as well as that other person.

Having a positive outlook on life is the first step to achieving success. You will never become a brilliant photographer if you keep telling yourself that it is impossible for you to capture something beautiful. What do you need to do instead? You need to be positive and think positive. Keep telling yourself that you can do it. Pessimism will bring you down every time it's OK to have doubts. But don't let your doubts get in the way of achieving success. Train your brain to have positive thoughts so that you can find a way out of these doubts. People like Michael Jordan and J.K. Rowling failed in their first attempts at that. They give up.

Instead, they kept their minds positive and kept striving. Now one of them is the most celebrated player in basketball, while the other is the creator of a world that every reader around the world loves. If they just told themselves that it's impossible for them to achieve something just because they failed the first time, would they have succeeded? Never. Attitude is the key to success. Your attitude matters a lot. If you're not serious about something, you can't expect to excel at it, can you? So you've made your mind about learning to play the piano to actually learn. You have to stay determined. There's no going back. Once you've made up your mind, keep reminding yourself that you are only stopping once you've made it possible.

Don't be lazy about something. If you've joined a piano class for learning, go to it regularly. Don't miss a class just because you don't feel like going or you're too lazy to go. Tell yourself that missing even one day will put you behind here. It's very important to not listen to others. People like to share their experiences, especially if they've had a hard time with it. Someone might tell you that you'll never learn because they themselves didn't manage to. If someone failed at something, that doesn't mean you will too. Maybe they did not have the dedication or positive outlook. You, on the other hand, have positivity and determination and you will succeed.

Most importantly, have faith in yourself. When you wake up everyday, tell yourself that it's possible for you to do it. Remind yourself of all the challenges that you've already overcome and prepare for the ones you're going to face. Think of a school or college. Everyone goes to the same place and has the same teachers, books and environment. So why is it that some of them manage to excel at studies while others don't? They must be doing something extra that others aren't. It's their attitude that takes them forward. They work extremely hard and they don't let anything stop them from getting what they want. This is what you need.

You don't let anything distract you or derail you. Learn to take a blow. Life isn't all cotton candy and unicorns. If you start a journey, you're bound to face bumps along the road. You must be prepared for everything. Keep your disaster management plan ready so that you aren't totally thrown off by any problem you face. Sometimes one thing can ruin an entire day or week. Learn to look at the brighter picture. Think of all the positive things that happened that day. A good way to do it is to keep a gratitude journal, write in it about everything that you are grateful for. So every time you're hit with a failure or a hurdle, read the journal to feel better. Problems are there to teach you something.

Every problem that you face along the way will help you polish your skills and nourish your personality. Don't lose hope just because one thing didn't go right. Learn from the mistakes you made and teach yourself how to do better next time. If you put your heart to a task, it can never be impossible. Always remember that there is no dead end. Sometimes when you are trying to do something, it might not be possible to do it with the first method. There are other ways to do that. If you have decided to read more often, don't be discouraged because books are too expensive. You can always go to a library or borrow books. Also, you can read books online or get PDFs easily, so don't treat your money issue as a dead end, change your direction and reach your goal.

A very popular quote teaches us that nothing is impossible because the word itself says that I'm possible. Keep this in mind. Every time you face a tragedy, it could be hard to stay positive if your environment's filled with negativity. Use positive words when you define your life or. Purpose. Spend time with people who will always push forward and encourage you rather than telling you to give up after the first blow, when you've learned how to channel your inner energy and keep your mind positive. You realize that nothing is impossible. Indeed, as you may know, it's only impossible until it is done. So do it and make it possible.

Live In The Moment

In this chapter, we'll talk about living in the moment. Living in the moment means to be fully aware and mindful of the present moment. It may involve some effort on your part, as it means not dwelling unnecessarily on the past or being overly anxious about the future. To live in the moment is to seize the moment you are in living it to the fullest, experiencing it without letting the past or the future distract you. In fact, living in the moment means acknowledging that someday will never come. If anything, it's already here. It's right now. So don't put off your goals just because it's not the right time or you don't have the funds. You can still work for your goals. Despite these setbacks, the time may never be right unless you're prepared for it.

So prepare right now. This presents the entire idea of living in the now and not just living it, but realizing the importance of it, giving it the emotions and thought that it rightfully demands, focusing on what you have now, focusing on the task at hand, and focusing on all that you can thank today for being present and mindful. Being present in the now and being mindful of the very moment you're living in allows you to make it even more valuable and meaningful instead of pondering over the past or worrying over the future. Make the most out of the present. If your goal is to spend more quality time with your family, then do so.

Say you're in a family gathering. But instead of giving family the attention they deserve the moment your eyes are glued to the phone screen, your ear is not paying attention to what the person sitting next to you is saying. You nod your head every once in a while without paying attention to what's been said at all. Even if the phone is put aside, the mind still remains occupied with it. The precious few hours you finally spare for the family time all go to waste and you have no clue when you'll be able to spare some time for them again. Instead, seize the moment, live it and be mindful of it. Make the most out of the opportunity at hand, not letting distractions take away what you have now.

Feel the moment and embrace it. Unless you learn to be present and mindful of the moment, you won't be able to give it your best first date, a late night call with your best friend. Walk with your dad. We do it all, but we don't give it our all. We're incomplete when all these moments slip through our fingers just because we were too busy being in so many places, states and moments in time to be actually present, we were too distracted to be present in the moment as a whole. Meditate. If you find yourself caving into distractions, consider meditation.

Meditation can be very helpful in learning how to live in the moment. It's a practice that helps find inner peace and acceptance, both of which are essential for being mindful of the present moment. It's also a great way to relax so that you're able to let go of all the stress, anxiety and thoughts of the past or future that haunt you. Unless you're truly relaxed, there is no living in the moment because the present gets overshadowed by the past or the future. Meditation techniques are preferably practiced in a serene, calm, natural environment.

Think of times are places like early morning, near a lake or in a field where there are no beeping phones, no honking cars, just the consistent melodic sound of water and the birds chirping meditation would require you to focus on these slowly tugging away at all the thoughts that had occupied your mind. It teaches you to live that very moment to the fullest, to be able to sense and appreciate it fully. Even breathing during meditation has a significant effect. Deep and relaxing breaths help you feel like you are taking in positive energy and getting rid of negativity. Burdening your mind with a couple of deep breaths.

You can feel the relaxation and peace take you over so you're able to enjoy these moments of peaceful solitude. Making a daily habit of meditation will help you stay calm and focused on the present moments throughout the day. Practice, gratitude, gratitude and living in the moment, go hand in hand without living in the moment, you can't be grateful for the little things that make life worth living. A witty answer, a hilarious joke, that first bite of a delicious steak, the pattern of rain against the window, the giggle of your child when he sees you. If you're not mentally present and mindful of these little things that make every moment of life precious, you can never be grateful.

How can you know the worth and value of these things if you're too lost in the past or worries of the future to live such moments when you live in the now, you experience each moment completely and you learn to appreciate it. Be happy with what you have now, with the contentment that where you are, who you are with, what you are doing is everything. The realization that what is in your hands right now is the best without thinking, hey, it would be better if this is good, but learn to be grateful for what you have without any ifs or buts. Don't waste away what you have by thinking of something you once had and lost, or by wishing for something you may never have.

Be grateful for what you're now, of constantly letting the past distract you, keeps you tied to it, keeps you from making the most of the present and constantly thinking of the future of what could be what could have been. All of these thoughts do not change what has happened and can't help you decide what happens in the future. What has already been and what will be are not in your control, but it is in your control to live in the moment, to enjoy the present, to live every moment in a way that makes it count. Measuring your success by what you have now is so much more than imagining what could have been or could be.

Being Adventurous

In this chapter, we'll discuss being adventurous. Being adventurous is to experience something different from the usual, something exciting and maybe even risky for every individual, the word adventure means different things. For some, it may just be staying up late and out past the curfew. For others, it could be skydiving. Everyone finds different things to be exciting and adventurous. Whatever it means to you as an individual, everyone should feel it often enough to make memories and to make life worth the while. Without adventure, the daily grind of life slowly strips away excitement and experiences that are important for the growth of a person. Adventures, contributing, keeping relationships from getting boring.

They contribute in letting you keep our personality from becoming dull. Step out of your comfort zone. Your comfort zone can be a very small, confined space in this small space. All things are familiar to you. There are no new experiences here, no new chapters to learn and no challenges. Stepping out of your comfort zone means trying new things that you're not comfortable or familiar with. Try doing things that you haven't done before or never thought you'd ever do. Push yourself to get new experiences, to get some excitement in life. Confining yourself to the comfort zone will never allow you to grow as a person.

Instead, it'll make you that person in a gathering who has no stories to tell. It'll make you that person no one invites to hang out anymore because you're not open to trying new things. And not to mention that it'll definitely stand in the way of achieving any success. It does not mean that you need to transform everything about you overnight. Rather, it is something you need to do for yourself once in a while. You can never enjoy doing the same things over and over. A little adrenaline rush never did any harm. Without stepping out of your comfort zone and being adventurous. You'll one day look back at life and see nothing but a plateau.

Adventures and things we do for excitement are the highs in life. The best and most joyful moments can never be experienced in that small, confined space we call a comfort zone. The fear of the unknown and unfamiliar can make it hard to do so. But once you learn to take little steps out of the comfort zone, you realize how the benefits far exceed the fears. And only after this will you be able to take big leaps out of the comfort zone and be adventurous. It'll help you learn more about yourself, about your strengths and weaknesses, be open minded and learn from experiences to enrich life with adventures. It's important to be open minded and to learn from experiences.

To be open minded is to accept that there are things you don't know about and also things that you could be wrong about. It means to be open to the idea of changing your thoughts, opinions and perceptions from new experiences and being open to new challenges and ideas. For example, a narrow minded person will always respond with a no when asked to join in. Anything exciting a pessimist would not only refuse, but also go on to explain all the things that could possibly go wrong. An open minded person, on the other hand, would be open to not only hearing about new ideas, but also trying out something new and adventurous.

It's the same as one ordering the same thing from the menu every time compared to the one trying out new items and cuisines. The latter will have far better experiences, some good and some bad. Every time you experience something new, there's something to be learned from that experience. Just as a traveler learns about the hospitality of people in a particular place, the different foods to try out there or the problems to be wary of. On the contrary, someone who is too afraid to invest so much time, energy and money on traveling and getting out of the comforts of home will learn nothing new from living each day, exactly the same as the previous prioritizing adventure over convenience and safety. However, this does not mean you risk your safety and security for adventure.

It doesn't mean putting your life or the life of others at stake. What it means instead is that you need to let yourself out of the shell that makes you feel safe, and that ease to prioritize adventure over convenience would mean that you're willing to go that extra mile to bring some excitement to your life. It's similar to what happens to a child with overprotective parents, one who isn't allowed to be friends with someone the parents have not approved of, not allowed to swing faster, not allowed to eat sweets, kept on tightly controlled schedules and so on. Compare him to a child whose parents are willing to let their child try new things, make new friends and learn from his own experiences. The personalities of these two will be totally opposite.

The former will always play by the rules, never learn to be independent, and never have the self-confidence to step out for an adventure. But the latter would know well that life is all about taking. Chances and learning from the outcomes, enjoying life through the adventure of it all, when you compare the two growth and success are almost always contrasted with comfort and safety, whereas growth leads to learning, creating, doing, resisting and failing. Comfort leads to stability, pleasure, protection and feeling good. But growth can't happen if you choose comfort over learning and success demands growing, overcoming obstacles, maybe even failing, but then getting up and trying again so you can't continue to keep clinging to the easy and avoiding what's challenging if you want to be successful at anything.

Words Of Success

In this chapter, we'll discuss words of success, words in languages that are unique to human beings only. They're like a superpower, which you can either use for the good or the bad. Unfortunately, people don't often realize the impacts words can have, whether it's the expression of love, the instructions on a manual or the speech of a captain just before a game. The words we use can change the outlook on everything. In fact, words probably linger longer in our memories than actual faces or whole events. So it's wise not to underestimate what words can do for yourself and for others. Beliefs are shaped from the words you use. Has someone ever passed a remark that makes you insecure till date? Things like you have a funny smile, you have a big nose, you have really bad breath leaving you with that insecurity for life so that you now always smile with a hand over your mouth or you get nervous speaking to someone too close to your face.

That's how words mold your beliefs. That's how words from others change what you think of yourselves. The same goes for compliments. It's surprising how a few words of appreciation can make you believe more in yourself. A simple color that looks so good on you will subconsciously always make you look for that color or words of appreciation from a teacher or mentor will encourage you to work harder and improve. This is exactly how words factor into success and failure. A common example of this is what you hear from a doctor, be it a serious disease or an aesthetic related problem. You hang on to every word that doctor tells you, not only the patient himself, but everyone related to him. Believe in the doctor's words religiously.

If the doctor speaks kindly and reassures the patient time and again that he will be cured, that this treatment is the best one, the patient will start feeling relaxed and better right away. If the doctor doesn't give any such reassurance and just hands over a prescription, the patient will stay restless and unsure about his treatment. Mind your vocabulary. The words you use can pave your way to success or downfall. Come to think of it, speakers make a living out of it, be it a religious speaker or a motivational speaker or a teacher. They all use their vocabulary to their best in order to convey things better to you, in order to improve your understanding of a concept and leave an impact on you.

When sitting through a job interview, you're basically being assessed on how you speak. The qualifications are all there on the resume, but the ability to communicate only comes through words. A candidate who sounds more convincing and capable has a higher chance of securing the job, even if others are more qualified. The right words are not only more convincing, but will also be an indicator of how well read you are for students. Vocabulary can make a huge difference. Without the right choice of words, it's very likely that they will fail to express how good their concepts are and might not do so well on a test. So mind your vocabulary as it can shape the level of your success. Even in relationships, vocabulary can save you, or in the other case, get you into trouble with the right words.

You can be more expressive of your feelings, good or bad, so that the other person knows exactly how you feel. It keeps things from getting boring and monotonous. Say your spouse wants to know how they look every time they dress up for you. Do not just stick with beauty every time. Use other expressions to tell them how you feel to boost their confidence and encourage them to put in that extra effort for you next time as well. And more importantly. So that is believable. Otherwise, they'll just think your words don't carry meaning at all. Use more I can rather than I can't. These are words that are entirely related to you, they can make you test your abilities or they can make you give up. Read a new recipe. That seems yummy, but too complicated was your answer. I can't do this.

Did you just tell yourself that without even trying? Can you ever hope to succeed at something if you don't even try? The more you use this phrase, the more opportunities of success you'll miss out on the ratio. How often you use I can or I can't can bring much more success and positivity in your life. I can symbolize all the risks you're willing to take, all the new things you're willing to try, all the chances you take, the faith you have in yourself, the limits that you establish for yourself and how much you're willing to push yourself to achieve what you want. I can't, on the other hand, symbolize the exact opposite.

It's all the chances you miss the times. You refuse to see if you could push past an obstacle, the opportunities that you didn't let yourself avail and basically failure without even a single try. Try making your choice of words positive using. I can so that you can reprogram your subconscious mind to believe things about yourself, your potential and your aspirations, because what you believe about yourself can have a real impact on the outcomes of events. It's in your own control. Which of these words you use for yourself.

Life-Long Learning

In this chapter, we'll talk about being a lifelong learner, learning is not limited to how many school and college years you've had. Instead, it's a constant ongoing process of evolution, one that involves acknowledging that you don't know everything. It's an important factor in shaping your personality, introducing new concepts and ideas to you and helping you educate yourself without any limitations. If anything, the worst thing you could do to yourself is insist that you already know everything. But choosing to evolve isn't always easy. Evolving means mastering success by continuously becoming a better version of your current self. It also implies that you'd be humble enough to accept correction and improvement, embrace learning and constant improvement in order to become the best version of yourself, you need to implement this rule in your life.

For this, you need to accept the fact that no information you have is already complete and there could be more to know about it. Be open to more knowledge and facts. Instead of being rigid and deciding that what you already know is final and enough, say you hear about a new research paper on one of the subjects you had while graduating. Not being open to constant improvements and knowledge would make you think I don't need to waste any time reading this. On the other hand, your approach to it could be as a lifelong learner, in which case you'll constantly struggle to further improve your learning and educate yourself.

Also, it's only at school that parents or teachers push you to study and learn whatever's in the curriculum. After that, you're on your own and learning becomes a self-motivated task. It's a personal choice you make every day that doesn't necessarily imply studying alone. Instead, it implies the overall education you have. You can learn from a documentary that is completely unrelated to your career. You can learn how to milk cows from a relative who owns a farm, or you can learn how to make jam from your grandmother. The point is just to learn from anywhere about anything, never stopping learning. There are so many reasons why you should never stop learning and not one logical reason why you shouldn't.

The struggle and desire to learn all your life can shape your personality for the better. Everyone knows that one person in their circle who's just so charismatic and interesting to talk to someone who genuinely has something to contribute to conversations instead of mere opinions, someone who has knowledge and stories to share with everybody. Such are lifelong learners. When someone decides to never stop learning, they also decide to be more independent, useful and hence successful. Learning also makes you more influential. It makes people consider your opinion and take whatever you say seriously because they know it comes from deep knowledge and is based on facts rather than intuition.

If anything, learning is the minimum requirement for success in any field or life in general. You need to keep increasing your knowledge to keep up with everything that's going on. If it's a specific field where you need to succeed, then you need to engage in some maintenance learning. This keeps you on track and keeps you from falling behind. If you need to groom yourself further, you need to get into some growth. Learning this type of learning expands the mind by teaching new skills you didn't have before. And finally, there's something called shock learning, which contradicts something that you knew before.

For the most part, this can potentially be the most beneficial type of learning as you first have to unlearn something that you knew before then you have to relearn the new information which gives you new insight into an old situation. Unfortunately, most people choose to ignore this in favor of the old information and sabotage their own success. You need to be never afraid of change. What stops you from becoming a lifelong learner? And the reason why most people fail to have this approach is because of themselves. After being done with a subject, most students never go back to the library to open up a new book about the same subject, same as the case. With all other situations in our lives, we are not open to learning.

If someone tries to get our facts right, we end up getting in an argument because we're too stubborn to admit that we could be wrong and the other person is actually doing us a favor. It's important to remember that the one thing that you're most short of in life is time. It can be a huge barrier to lifelong learning. In order to be a lifelong learner, you need to change your mindset and concepts about it. You need to make learning a priority. There are no rules, no boundaries. You need to embrace this journey and learn about anything from anyone or anywhere. It's not about pouring yourself into books. It's about things you learn every day from those around you. It's not.

Confined to the walls of a lecture hall live as if you were going to die tomorrow, learn as if you were to live forever, Mahatma Gandhi, great thinkers, leaders and influencers all had many things in common. Lifelong learning is one of them. In order to achieve personal success and also to be more valuable and useful to those around you. Be a lifelong learner. Don't confine your learning to years or places, don't confine yourself to learning just from books. Anyone, in any event can teach you important things as long as you set your mind to it. Have a strong desire, almost a hunger for knowledge without real passion towards learning. It'll be like a burden you bear in school years, not education.

No Such Thing As Failure

In this chapter, we'll talk about, there's no such thing as failure in life, you are bound to go through some ups and downs. A strong person is one who manages to pull through anything and everything to be strong and win in life. It's important to remember that there's no such thing as failure. Don't be afraid of rejection. The idea of failure is different for everyone. For some people, the idea is quite daunting, while for others it's just downright depressing and discouraging. Failure comes in different forms and through different means. Sometimes it's disguised as your inability to excel at something and others. It comes as rejection. Rejections can be a huge blow.

If you're not prepared for it, you must always be prepared for rejection because it will come your way at some point in time. Don't be afraid of it and don't refuse to accept that it has come your way. Instead, accept it and polish yourself to be better. If you've been rejected from a college or co curricular program, ask yourself why it went wrong. Instead of being afraid of the idea, embrace it and use it to make yourself better. Everyone develops a fear of failure as they grow older. It's easy to see because young people have less fear of failure than older ones. As an infant, you learned how to walk through failure. You tried to get up, but you fell down.

But did you stop trying altogether? No. You went through the whole process of trial and error to learn how to walk perfectly. The same principle applies to your adult life. Sometimes rejection hurts your self-esteem. But if you think of it as feedback rather than a failure, when things are much better, treat your rejection as feedback and find ways to enhance yourself. Most importantly, don't let the fear of rejection stop you from trying at all. At least give something one or two attempts, if not more. With the right amount of dedication, you will be able to achieve whatever you want. Failures are stepping stones for success.

It's quite a paradox that you have to fail in order to succeed. Yet it makes a lot of sense. If you fail at something that doesn't make you a failure, it just makes you a person who's learned something from their attempt. A world renowned example of this is Thomas Edison performing about 10000 experiments to come up with the perfect model for a light bulb. What kept him going after his first or hundredth try failed the determination to succeed. He didn't treat the futile experiments as failures. Instead, he treated them as 10000 new things that he learned. There are many examples from history which show that failure is essential in the journey to success.

You can't really expect to learn something if your path is obstacle free, can you? But when you fail, you see your mistakes and that gives you a chance to refine yourself. This is why all successful people are so refined in their ways and choices they've learned from failures in life. Michael Jordan, the famous basketball star, admits that he's only successful because he failed over and over again. You might think that failure would only break your hopes and dim the lights along the road. Yet this isn't entirely true. It just depends on how you decide to see something. As a first time parent, you might think that you're failing every time something goes wrong.

Think of it this way. Every time you do something wrong, there's something you learn not to do in the future. With time you get better and parenting becomes much easier with your second child. As long as you learn from the experience, it's a success. Failure is an amazing experience in its own way. When you fail, you learn new things about yourself. You learn a new way to cope with something, and you discover your capabilities that never surfaced before. Just like that. You also learn new things about the task at hand. It's perhaps not possible to learn as much from success because it comes with perfection. But there's so much that you can learn from failure as it gives you a chance to grow as a person.

You only fail if you give up. As long as you keep trying, you're not failing. If your own failures seem overwhelming, then learn from the experience of successful people. They have a habit of never giving up. Instead of gloating over their failures, they use them to their advantage and pave their way to success. They've all taught us that it's OK to fall and that there's no shame in making this fall your strength and getting up with more determination and force that is unbeatable. Always remember your failure isn't a stop sign. Might be a sign for you to change your direction or be more focused on the one you're already heading to. But in no way is it a stop sign. If you stop, that's when you fail. As long as you keep going on and becoming better, you're succeeding. Never let others force you into believing that you're a failure.

It's your journey. And you know how far you have come. You. We just need to learn from every experience, and that'll soon lead you to success. Everyone faces setbacks in life, but it's people who experiment and persist that become successful later in life. You might have failed multiple times to keep your blog or website running. If you learn from each failure and rectify every mistake you made, you'll have your passion fulfilled in no time. It's only you who determines that you have failed, not your circumstances, nor the people around you. Not everyone gets to play easy in life. Hurdles are bound to come your way. But remember what Tony Robbins says. There's no such thing as failure. There are only results.

Recap

In the end, the formula to achieving success isn't all that complicated. It's within your grasp once you've decided to go after it with everything you've got by following these principles that help you solve problems, overcome frustrations, develop patience, boost self-esteem and improve yourself as a person, you can be sure that you will be successful in improving the overall quality of life.

Healthy Eating Lifestyle

In this chapter, you're going to learn how to make eating a healthy lifestyle and not a duty, basically a healthy diet is the basis for a well functioning body. It's an important part of leading a healthy lifestyle. Food is the source of energy for all of our bodily functions and directly affects how our bodies and minds function in every stage of life. There are several details that are involved in eating healthy, including moderation, variety and balance. Now a person should try to balance different nutrients and food like protein, food, vegetables, dairy products and grains while minimizing alcohol, processed food and saturated fats. And I bet that you didn't know that eating a variety of food from each food group helps a person to get all of the important nutrients. Healthy eating helps to prevent conditions like heart disease, hypertension, diabetes and some types of cancer.

Protein helps in repairing body tissues while carbohydrates provide the body with energy, therefore making healthy eating a habit that will go a long way in ensuring the health of an individual. But remember this. It shouldn't be a duty to eat healthy. It should be adopted as a constant lifestyle. Generally, we all know the benefits of having a healthy body. But however, a lot of people don't really know how to obtain and sustain a healthy body. That's where the real challenge is. But did you know that many of the sicknesses and diseases that we see today are the result of indifferent or ignorant attitudes towards necessary self care, poor eating habits and always thinking that it won't happen to me? Well, just think about this. How many patients can foresee that they're going to get sick? Because most of the time when it hits them, it's already too late.

There's a golden old saying of an ounce of prevention is worth a pound of cure. A high percentage of people can have preventable diseases if they have sufficient and accurate knowledge on nutrition and supplements, the key to a balanced diet is to eat in moderation. It is an important tip to eating healthily. Eating in moderation is a way of life, not a way of dieting. If you choose to practice this health, you may just find a new sense of confidence and awareness of yourself and your body. Now you can choose which path you wish to take to make your life's journey a fulfilling, joyful and healthy one. Start by making today healthier than yesterday.

But you're probably asking, how can I do that? Well, number one, you set achievable goals. These are goals that are going to gradually change your health status and overall lifestyle into a better and healthier one. You're going to see and feel the difference once you start working on achieving these goals in a timely manner. No, to begin with cultivating the right mindset that will fuel your willpower to stay on track, but also changes your daily mood to strive for the better. It is extremely essential that you learn to feel good about what you're doing and how you're going to transform.

And finally, number three, always think to yourself that you look good because it increases your self-esteem. If you look at people who are struggling with mental disorders related to eating habits, let's say anorexia, where they refused to eat or maybe even bulimia nervosa, also known as binge eating, you're going to see the mental pattern falls into the same category, which they think that they're not good enough. But the truth is, it's a mental illness that leads an individual to problematic eating disorders that harm one's overall health and lifestyle. And it can be life threatening as well. Therefore, it's super important to have a positive mindset about your own body and how you see yourself.

Now, let me ask you a question. What do you know about mindset now? I'm sure you've heard about how mindset plays the biggest role in determining your actions. And yes, it is indeed true. Your mindset is the fuel to your actions. When you feel good about yourself, you will look good. And you might not be good enough now. But don't worry, don't beat yourself up. All you have to do is to keep a positive mindset. And not just that. A fitter and healthier you leads to higher productivity as well. And the truth is, most people think that a diet is associated with weight loss, bodybuilding and good body shapes. But what they forgot is that a diet is equally important in overall health and well-being.

By taking the time to learn how to eat healthy, you've stepped onto the route that leads to an in shape, healthy body. And finally, take a minute to think over this famous quote. Success is a journey, not a destination. Now take that quote and replace the word success with the word fitness. Learning how to make the correct decisions in your nutrition will convert to a healthy lifestyle that's never ending. Begin to construct the habits that will step up your enjoyment and quality of life today.

Powerful Benefits of Eating Healthy

In this chapter, you'll learn about all of the benefits and eating healthy. Now, before we get to the benefits of eating healthy, let me ask you a question. Did you know that eating nutritiously is one of the most important things you can do to enhance and maintain your health? A healthy diet can balance out your body and allow it to function in its most efficient state. Eating nutritionally balanced meals helps the body to work to its full potential, which is particularly important for people living with busy and tight schedules, or just people who are constantly feeling not energized and easily falling sick.

Many people find that they can improve their quality of life and sense of well-being simply by focusing on the aspects of health that can be controlled and changed like a healthy diet as well as healthy eating can also stop or slow down the advancement of numerous chronic illnesses like heart disease and diabetes, osteoporosis and a few types of cancer. Eating healthy can also help you deal better with both physical and mental strain operations and even the common cold or influenza. Now let's talk about the fundamentals of healthy living. One consumes an assortment of nutritious foods to eat in moderation. Three size matters.

So limit your portions. Eating healthy can promote a lot of benefits to your body and also your life in general. When we eat the right kind of food, we are allowing the body to be properly nourished. Hence, as a result, we will be able to gain health benefits from our healthful efforts. There are five benefits all together which include that it can improve your immune system. It enhances your mood, your mental health, your energy, and you live longer. Number one, it can improve your immune system.

Good nutrition is essential to a strong immune system which may offer protection from seasonal illness like the flu and other health problems, including cancers, arthritis, abnormal cell development and allergies. A lot of sickness can be prevented if the right precaution is taken to help protect yourself against infection and boost your immunity by including these nutrients into your eating plan. With a strong immune system, you're going to feel constantly boosted with energy and strength to carry out daily activities. No, to enhance your mood. And not just that eating healthy can have a positive impact on your life by leading to a more sustained, elevated mood. Oh, and it can reduce stress as well.

A healthy cognitive system is essential to regulating mood, and certain nutrients have a profound impact on maintaining normal brain function. When your body is in a chronic state of stress, it breaks down protein to prepare for battle. But certain foods have the ability to moderate the body's level of cortisol. The stress hormone. Number three, boost your mental health. Nutrition is a key contributor to good mental health. It is one of the most obvious yet under-recognized factors in the development of major trends in mental health. Food plays an important contributing role in the development, management and prevention of specific mental health problems like schizophrenia, depression and attention deficit hyperactivity disorder, as well as Alzheimer's disease. Here are five foods that keep the mind working at its best: lean protein, leafy greens, fatty fish, wholegrain yogurt with active cultures. Number four boosts your energy. Eating the right nutritive food can also boost your energy levels, making you prepared to face each day.

Food can boost energy by supplying calories, by pushing your body to burn more calories more efficiently, and in some cases by delivering caffeine. When you have an energized body and clear mind, it also increases our brain power. Eating healthy food can ensure you to achieve a balanced nutrition that can help to regulate your brain activity, to fuel your mental power that will get you through your busiest days. Five Live longer. Did you know that emerging nutrition science research, as well as data collected from people in their 90s and beyond shows what, when and how we eat has a profound influence on how long we live around the world. Certain groups of people enjoy exceptionally long lives.

Consider the lucky people of Okinawa. These Pacific Islanders have an average life expectancy of more than 81 years, compared to 78 in the United States and the worldwide average of just 67. A diet rich in fruits and vegetables, high in nutrients and low in calories is your best bet for a long life. It is vital for your health and maintenance. Some of the foods include broccoli, grapes, salad, avocado, olive oil, berries and beans, along with grains and seeds, less red meat, fish, bananas and organic food.

Alkaline Foods vs Acidic

In this chapter, we're going to talk about alkaline foods versus acidic foods before going into detail. First, you have to understand that food can be classified into two groups, namely the acidic food group and the alkaline food group. Now, the question is, why are these foods categorized as such? The answer is because they affect the urine level when they're consumed. Our bodies' acid alkaline balance, also known as P.H., can affect our overall well-being. Whatever food we consume, once it enters into our body, it will undergo processing and become acidic. Too much acid consumption can deplete the minerals in our body, thus growing the risk of heart disease, kidney problems and osteoporosis. That's why we need alkaline food as well. It helps to balance out the acidity in our body. Next, we'll talk about P value.

P stands for power of hydrogen. It's a measure of the acidity or alkalinity of our bodies, fluids and tissues. The total scale ranges from one to 14, with seven considered to be neutral. Our ideal is slightly alkaline, seven point three to seven point four or five. If the body value is below seven, that means it's acidic, whereas if it's above seven, it's alkaline. Now let's talk about the most common form of imbalance. The most common form of imbalance is excess acidity.

It can lead to numerous health issues and it can even be life threatening and acidic can occur from an acid forming diet, toxic overload, emotional stress, immune reactions, or any process that deprives the cells of oxygen and other nutrients.

Assuming if the reach is acidic, the body will try to compensate for it using the alkaline minerals. If the diet doesn't contain enough minerals to compensate a buildup of acids in the cells will occur. A healthy body maintains adequate alkaline reserves to balance the acids in order to maintain this.

Why do you think acidosis is more common in our society? The reason acidosis is more common in our society is mostly due to the typical human diet, which is far too high in acid producing animal products, things like meat, eggs and dairy, and far too low in alkaline producing foods like fresh vegetables. In addition to this, we consume acid producing processed foods like white flour, sugar and drink, acidic producing beverages like coffee and soft drinks. We use too many drugs which are acid forming, and we use artificial chemical sweeteners like NutraSweet Spoonful, Sweet'N Low, equal or even aspartame, which are poisonous and extremely acid forming.

Now that we've already covered the reason for acidosis, let's move on to talk about its consequences. If these mineral losses and metabolic abnormalities continue, we can increase our risk for a number of conditions, including premature aging, osteoporosis, weaker brittle bones, fractures and bone spurs, mood swings, low energy and chronic fatigue, slow digestion and elimination. Bladder and kidney conditions, including kidney stones, weight gain, obesity and diabetes. Slow metabolism and the inability to lose weight. Chronic inflammation, high blood pressure, weakened immunity. One of the best methods we can do to correct an overly acidic body is to clean up the diet and the lifestyle to maintain health.

The optimum diet should consist of 60 percent alkaline forming food and 40 percent acid forming food to restore health. The diet should consist of 80 percent alkaline forming food and 20 percent acid forming food. Generally, alkaline forming food consists of most fruits, green vegetables, spices, lentils, seasonings or herbs and seeds and nuts. Whereas acid forming food comprises meat, fish, poultry, eggs, grains and legumes. The alkaline diet is also known as the alkaline ash diet, or acid alkaline diet. It emphasizes alkaline foods such as fruits, vegetables and certain whole grains, which are low in caloric density. Healthy alkaline diet food involves the ideal balance between acidifying and alkaline foods.

Having an alkaline diet may have some potential in reducing morbidity as well as mortality from chronic diseases. Here is a list of some alkalis vegetables, spinach. It's very low in alkaline. It's moderate and alkaline with a seven point five to eight point zero. And spinach content raises alkalinity cabbage, low alkaline forming food with a moderate alkaline level of point seven five 2.8 zero. It's also a good substitute for coca and it's mineral rich. Sellery is a very low alkaline forming food. It's moderate alkaline level, has a seven point five to eight point zero, and it elevates acid food, 5.0 in alkaline direction, capsaicin or bell peppers, low alkaline forming food with a moderate alkaline level of seven point five to eight point zero.

It's a good substitute for coca and it's mineral rich. A list of alkalis, fruits, lemons, they're highly alkaline forming with a pair of eight point five to nine point zero and an excellent remedy against colds, coughs, sore throats, heartburn and gastric upsets. Limes are also extremely alkaline, forming foods with a level of eight point five to nine point zero and they purify the kidneys. Grapes are a very low alkaline forming food with a moderate alkaline level of seven point five to eight point zero and bananas. They're a very low alkaline forming food with a moderate alkaline level of seven point five to eight point zero. And they also elevate the acid food of five point zero in alkaline direction.

Understanding The Food Pyramid

In this chapter, you'll learn everything about the food pyramid without further ado, let's get started. So what exactly is the food pyramid? Well, it's a simple visual guide to the types and proportions of food that we should eat every day for good health. Food that contains the same type of nutrients are grouped together on each of the shelves of the food pyramid. This gives you a choice of different foods from which to choose a healthy diet. Using a food pyramid is a tool to follow different dietary guidelines and is a good start in the right direction. It will help you to get the right balance of nutritious food within your calorie range. Now will further elaborate on the different layers of the food pyramid.

There are three layers of the food pyramid, which include one, the foundation layer to the middle layer and three, the top layer. Now let's have a look at the foundation layer. The foundation layer includes the three plant based food groups, which are fruits, grains, vegetables and legumes. This layer makes up the largest portion of the pyramid at around 70 percent of what we should eat. Plant food should make up the largest portion of our diet plant. Food contains a wide variety of nutrients like vitamins, minerals and antioxidants. They're also the main source of carbohydrates and fiber in our diet.

A significant convergence of evidence suggests that plant based diets can help prevent and even reverse some of the top killer diseases in the Western world and can be more effective than medication and surgery. Older children, teens and adults should aim to have at least two servings of fruit and five servings of vegetables or legumes each day from the grains food group. We should choose mostly whole grains like quinoa, oats and brown rice and wholemeal, whole grain, high cereal, fiber varieties of bread, crisp breads, pasta and cereal foods or over highly processed, refined varieties. Now we move on to the middle layer. This layer includes yogurt, cheese, milk and alternatives and lean meat, fish, eggs and legumes.

Food groups, food in the Milk, Yogurt, Cheese and Alternatives group primarily provides us with calcium and protein, plus other vitamins and minerals. This food group also refers to non-dairy options like soy rice or cereal milks, which have at least 100 milligrams per 100 milliliters of added calcium chews. Reduced fat options of these foods to limit excess kilojoules from saturated fat food in the lean meats, poultry, fish, eggs, nuts, seeds and legumes. S. are our main sources of protein. This food group is rich in protein and is also a good source of other nutrients like iodine, iron, zinc and vitamins, especially some B group vitamins. The animal food in this group also contains vitamin B 12, and some of them contain omega three fatty acids.

Now we'll look at the top layer. This layer refers to healthy fats that we need small amounts of every day to support heart health and brain function. The top level of the food pyramid consists of your non-essential foods like fats, oil and sweet. This is the only level of the pyramid that should be restricted. There are no serving guidelines for this level and you should generally try to avoid foods that are high in fat or sugar. You should choose food that contains healthy fats instead of food that contains saturated fats and trans fat chews on refined polyunsaturated and monounsaturated fats from plant sources like extra virgin olive oil nuts and seed oils to limit the amount of saturated fat that you consume and avoid trans fat. We also get healthy fats from food and other food groups such as seeds, avocados, fish and nuts.

We need these healthy fats to support our health and brain function, healthy eating guidelines. The shape of the food pyramid immediately suggests that some foods are good and some should be eaten more often, but also that others aren't so good and should only be eaten occasionally. The layers represent major food groups that contribute to the total diet. But how do you link them together? One chooses water to increase herbs and spices. Three limit your salt and added sugar to limit sodium and five limit added sugar water. Water is one of the most essential elements to health. A mere two percent drop in our bodies. Water supply can trigger signs of dehydration.

A healthy, sedentary adult living in a temperate climate should drink at least one and a half liters of water per. This level of water intake balances water loss and helps in keeping the body properly hydrated, the water you consume through food and drinks follows a very precise route to arrive in your cells, of which it is a vital constituent. Therefore, choose water as your main drink and avoid sugary options like soft drinks, sports drinks and energy drinks, increase herbs and spices. The use of herbs and spices has been incredibly important throughout history. Many were celebrated for their medicinal properties well before culinary use.

If you're looking to round out your healthy lifestyle, you'll want to stock up on the following herbs and spices and use them generously in your cooking or use them on their own to enhance the absorption and benefits received. Some of the best examples are arrowroot cinnamon, turmeric, basil, mint, cayenne, dill, weed and seed and curry powder limit salt in added sugar. The food pyramid reminds us to limit our intake of salt and added sugar. This means avoiding adding salt or sugar to food when we're cooking or eating and avoiding packaged foods and drinks that have salt or added sugar in the ingredients.

Some suggestions that can help you reduce your salt and sugar dependency include eating more home cooked meals, choosing frozen over, canned or delaying and salting. Even reducing these by small amounts can make us healthier. And last but not least, there are five stages of change that have been conceptualized for a variety of problem behaviors. Each of these stages describes an individual's attitude toward behavior change. Trying to change behavior before one is ready usually results in failure to develop new healthy behaviors. Small steps are the best bet for long term results.

These five stages include pre contemplation, contemplation, preparation, action and maintenance, pre contemplation, the stage at which there is no intention to change behavior in the immediate or foreseeable future. Many individuals in this state are unaware or under aware of their problems. They may not be ready to change a good strategy, assess knowledge, attitudes and beliefs and provide information to build on the existing knowledge, contemplation, the stage in which people are aware that a problem exists and are seriously thinking about overcoming it, but have not yet made a commitment to change or take any action. Making the leap from thinking about change to taking action can be hard.

Asking yourself about the pros or the benefits and the cons or the things that get in the way of changing your habits may be helpful. A good strategy is to discuss your motivation and barriers to change and your possible solutions. If you're in the preparation stage, you are about to take action to get started. Look at your list of pros and cons. How can you make a plan and move to action? Here's a good strategy. Assist in developing an action plan for change. Provide direction and encouragement. Action the stage in which individuals modify their behavior, experiences or their environment in order to overcome their problems.

Action involves the most overt behavioral changes and requires a considerable commitment of time and energy. A good strategy, reinforce decisions for change, offer continued support and reinforcement for positive changes. Maintenance knows that healthy eating and physical activity has become part of your routine. You need to keep things interesting, avoid slip ups and find ways to cope with what life throws at you. A good strategy. Add variety and stay motivated. Mix up your routine with new activities, physical activity, buddies, recipes, rewards and food.

Food Cholesterol

In this chapter, we're going to talk about food, cholesterol, so what exactly is cholesterol? Cholesterol is a waxy substance which is made in the body by the liver, but it's also found in some food that we eat in our daily lives. This soft, waxy substance is not only found in your bloodstream, but also in every cell in your body where it helps to produce cell membranes, hormones, vitamin D and bile acids that help you digest fat. However, having too much cholesterol in the blood can increase your risk of getting heart and circulatory diseases. But where does cholesterol come from? Cholesterol comes from your body as well as from what you eat.

Now there is about 75 percent of cholesterol that's made by your body and the amount is determined by your family history. So the remaining 25 percent of cholesterol comes from what you eat. The cholesterol level in your blood will increase if you eat food with saturated fats and trans fat. There are two main types of blood cholesterol. One is low density lipoprotein and two is high density lipoprotein, low density lipoprotein, also known as the bad cholesterol, because it develops plaque which will clog the arteries and make them less flexible. It collects in the walls of your blood vessels where it can cause blockages. Higher LDL levels puts you at greater risk for a heart attack or stroke due to the narrowed artery when the clot is formed.

This condition is called atherosclerosis. High density lipoprotein, also known as good cholesterol, helps to discard the bad cholesterol away from the arteries and back to the liver to break it down and pass the cholesterol from the body. In other words, HDL reduces reuses and recycles LDL cholesterol by transporting it to the liver where it can be reprocessed. So you will be protected from heart attacks and strokes when you have a healthy level of HDL cholesterol. Remember, you're not alone. About one hundred million other Americans have high cholesterol. High cholesterol comes from a variety of sources, including your family history and what you eat here is a visual journey through the most common causes.

Some of the most common causes of high blood cholesterol include your diet, your activity level, your age and gender, genetics and cigarette smoking. A diet high in cholesterol, saturated fats and trans fats can raise blood cholesterol levels and puts you at risk for heart disease. You will find this unhealthy fat in food that comes from animals. Beef, pork, milk, butter, veal, milk, cheese and eggs contain saturated fat. Packaged food that contains palm oil, coconut oil or cocoa butter may have a lot of saturated fat. You will also find saturated fat and sticks of margarine, vegetable shortening and most cookies, crackers, chips and other snacks.

Your activity level, if your cholesterol numbers aren't where they should be working out, should be a key part of your get healthy strategy. By increasing your activity level, it will help you to lose or maintain your weight. Being overweight tends to increase the amount of low density lipoprotein in your blood, the kind of lipoprotein that's been linked to heart disease, whether you're a male or female. As you get older, your risk for heart disease increases dramatically. For instance, a 62 year old man is 500 times more likely than a 22 year old man to die from heart disease in the next year. In men, cholesterol levels generally level off after the age of 50.

In women, cholesterol levels stay fairly low until menopause, after which they rise to about the same level as men. Your family history may also affect your cholesterol level. High cholesterol may run in your family. If family members have or had high cholesterol, you may also have it. There are over 100 genes that can affect blood fats and how these are metabolized in the body. Sometimes just one faulty gene is enough to increase your cholesterol to dangerous levels, and sometimes high cholesterol results from the small effects of many genes.

Some people will have high cholesterol even if they follow a healthy, balanced diet, low in saturated fats and trans fat. These people may need to take cholesterol lowering medicine as prescribed by their doctor. Cigarette smoking lowers your level of HDL or good cholesterol. It also injures the lining of the blood vessels and increases the risk of developing blood clots, which contributes to death, which contributes to arthroscopy. Neurosis or the hardening of the arteries damages the walls of your blood vessels, making them more likely to accumulate fatty deposits, even inhaling second hand cigarette smoke has been shown to lower HDL cholesterol.

And now the top five tactics to improve your cholesterol level lifestyle changes can help reduce cholesterol, keep you off cholesterol lowering medications, or enhance the effect or enhance the effect of your medications. Here are five lifestyle changes to get you started. One, eat heart healthy food to increase your physical activity. Three, lose weight. Four, drink alcohol only in moderation. Five, quit smoking. Even if you have years of unhealthy eating under your belt, making a few changes in your diet can reduce cholesterol and improve your heart health. Therefore, replace foods that are high in saturated fat with healthier options that can lower blood cholesterol levels and improve lipid profiles.

Exercise can improve cholesterol. Moderate physical activity can help raise high density lipoprotein or HDL cholesterol. The good cholesterol. The best plan for reducing your risk of cardiovascular disease is a combination of aerobic or cardio and resistance training. Spend an average of 40 minutes of moderate to vigorous intensity aerobic activity three to four times a week to improve cholesterol levels, as well as lower your blood pressure and risk for stroke and heart attack for overall cardiovascular health. Spend at least 150 minutes of moderate exercise or 75 minutes of vigorous exercise per week.

You can mix up moderate and vigorous activity if you'd like to stay motivated, find an exercise buddy or join an exercise group. And remember, any activity is helpful. Even taking the stairs instead of the elevator or doing a few sit ups while watching television can make a difference. Examples of moderate intensity exercise include ballroom dancing, playing, tennis, general gardening or bicycling. Examples of vigorous intensity exercise include hiking uphill or with a heavy backpack, swimming laps, jogging, race, walking or running, aerobic dancing or bicycling. If you've already implemented the first two strategies correctly, diet and exercise numbers on the scale may already be dropping, if not make a concerted effort to lose weight.

Since studies show that you may be able to reduce cholesterol levels significantly by losing five percent to 10 percent of your body weight for long term success with weight loss, the Mayo Clinic suggests making small, sustainable changes slowly incorporate physical activity into your daily routine in simple ways, such as brisk walking or doing simple house chores. Bring a healthy lunch from home instead of eating out, it all adds up. All of these can have a big impact on your weight, which could help lower your cholesterol. You should only drink alcohol in moderation. Moderate use of alcohol has been linked with higher levels of HDL cholesterol.

A few studies have found that people who drink alcohol in moderation have lower heart disease and might even live longer than those who abstain. Alcohol has also been tied to a lower risk of blood clots and decreased levels of inflammation markers. Too much alcohol can lead to serious health problems, including stroke, high blood pressure and heart failure. Quit smoking. The most well-documented impact that smoking has on cholesterol is how it lowers levels of high density lipoprotein or HDL. Smoking makes all heart health indicators worse. It causes inflammation not just in your lungs, but throughout your entire body, which can contribute to atherosclerosis, blood clots and risk of heart attack. If you smoke, quitting might improve your HDL cholesterol level. Studies have shown that HDL levels often go up soon after a person quits smoking.

Recommended Foods For Exceptional Health

In this chapter, we're going to talk about what are the recommended foods that we should consume to provide the best nutrients for our bodies. Now, why is it so important to eat the right food? Eating the right food means providing your body with the right amount of nutrition, and you can do it with a proper meal that is healthy while not trying to deprive yourself from other food to top things off. You can eat right and exercise regularly to achieve a well-balanced, healthy mind and body. Consuming food from a wide variety of sources helps maintain a healthy and interesting diet to ensure your body has the nutrients it needs to help reduce the risk of disease.

The best food choices include vegetables, fruits, whole grain, dietary fiber, healthy carbohydrates, calcium and healthy fats. Now let's talk about vegetables. One of the first best food choices is vegetables. I'm sure that each and every one of us knows the importance of vegetables in our daily diet. But do we really know why it's so useful in reducing weight? You may not know. So without further ado, let's begin. Vegetables are useful in reducing weight as they provide bulk and give a feeling of being full. And furthermore, the Balkan water count aides in the treatment of constipation to get the best out of vegetables they should be taking raw or just slightly cooked by steaming, boiling, broiling or stewing.

Green leafy vegetables provide a source of many nutrients, including iron fiber, vitamins, A and C, and potassium, which helps to purify the blood, heal the intestinal tract anemia and reduce the risk of developing diabetes. A good example of green vegetables are spinach, cabbage and broccoli, where they are best served after being steamed or lightly boiled. Red and yellow vegetables like tomatoes, pumpkin, eggplant, potato, carrot, beetroot, bitter gourd, are rich in nutrients and bitter gourds are rich in nutrients as well. They contain vitamin A, vitamin B, iron, potassium, calcium and fiber, which can improve body immunity and help to boost the body's metabolism.

Now, let's talk about fruits, fruits provide nutrients vital for health and the maintenance of your body. People who eat fruit as part of an overall healthy diet generally have a reduced risk of chronic diseases. The healthiest choices are fresh fruits or frozen without added sweeteners, as the sugar from fruits or fructose can be quite high. Fruit is naturally low in calories, fat and sodium and rich in folate, vitamin C, potassium and fiber. Some high potassium fruits include bananas, peaches, oranges, honey, do and cantaloupe. The fiber in fruit helps to lower cholesterol, and it protects against heart disease. Vitamin C and food like strawberries and citrus help with wound healing and keep gums and teeth healthy. Now let's talk about wholegrain eating. More whole grains is an easy way to add a layer of health insurance to your life.

Whole grains are better sources of fiber and other important nutrients like magnesium, selenium, potassium, protein, antioxidants, fiber, B vitamins and iron. Whole grains have been shown to reduce the risk of heart disease by lowering blood pressure and cholesterol levels along with blood coagulation. Whole grains have also been found to reduce the risks of many types of cancer. Fiber is important for healthy bowel function as it helps to reduce constipation and diverticular diverticulitis.

B vitamins help the body release energy from carbohydrates, fat and protein. Iron is used to carry oxygen in the blood. Selenium is important for a healthy immune system, and magnesium is a mineral used in building bones and releasing energy from muscles. Some of the healthy whole grains include whole wheat, oatmeal, quinoa, brown rice and whole grain, barley and corn. Now on to dietary fiber. Dietary fiber has many health benefits. Consuming foods which are high in fiber can reduce your risk of heart diseases. Stroke, diabetes, some cancers as well as losing weight. Foods that are high in fiber are usually derived from natural and unprocessed food. Good sources of fiber can be found in nuts, barley, whole grains, oatmeal, wheat, cereals and beans for vegetables.

They can be found in celery, carrots and tomatoes, whereas for fruits it can be found in berries, apples, pears and citrus fruits. It is best to start your day off with whole grain cereals or include unprocessed wheat bran into your preferred cereal to increase your fiber intake. Now we'll discuss healthy carbohydrates. Carbohydrates are an essential part of a healthy diet. Carbohydrates provide the body with glucose, which is converted to energy use to support bodily functions and physical activity. Most carbohydrates are naturally occurring in plant based foods such as grains.

Food manufacturers also add carbohydrates to processed foods in the form of starch or added sugar. Some of the common sources of naturally occurring carbohydrates include grains, milk, nuts, seeds, vegetables and fruits. Carbohydrate quality is important. Some types of carbohydrate rich foods are better than others. The healthiest sources of carbohydrates, unprocessed or minimally processed whole grains, vegetables, fruits and beans promote good health by delivering fiber, vitamins, minerals and a host of important phytonutrients. Now on to calcium. Calcium is important for overall health. It also plays an important role in muscle contraction, transmitting messages through the nerves and the release of hormones. Almost every cell in our body uses calcium in some way.

Our body requires calcium to maintain healthy bones and teeth. Dairy products are a good source of calcium, which they are also easily digested and absorbed into the body, like milk, unsweetened yogurt and cheese, vegetables like kale, romaine lettuce, celery, broccoli, fennel, green beans, cabbage, summer squash, Brussels sprouts and asparagus as well as criminy. Mushrooms are rich sources of calcium. Moreover, beans like black beans, white beans, pinto beans, kidney beans, black eyed peas or even baked beans are excellent. Choices for gaining calcium protein provides us the energy for our body to work, and overconsumption of protein can be detrimental to our kidneys. Fish, chicken or plant based proteins like beans, nuts and soy are the ones that contain high quality protein. Now let's talk about healthy fats.

People are often concerned about excess dietary fat, but. Not getting enough good fats may also cause health problems, eating fat can be heart healthy if you pick the right kind. The fat that we consume is digested and either used for energy stored in fat tissues or incorporated into other body tissues and organs. Fats exert powerful effects within the body. We need adequate fat to support metabolism, the health of various body tissues, immunity, cell signaling, hormone production and the absorption of many nutrients like vitamins and having enough fat will also help keep you feeling full between meals. Here are some examples of high fat foods that are actually incredibly healthy and nutritious foods like avocados, almonds, fatty fish, hazelnuts, cheese, dark chocolate, pecans, pumpkin seeds and sesame seeds.

Cooking Simple Healthy Meals

In this chapter, we're going to talk about cooking up some simple, healthy meals. When it comes down to feeding your body and mind, nothing is superior to preparing your food from scratch with quality ingredients and served with love. Now, have you ever wondered why it's so important to prepare your meals at home? This is because by doing so, it allows you to control the amount of salt, oil and other things that you use in your recipes. This, in turn, reduces the possibility of clogged arteries and weight gain. And not just that. Taking the time to plan your weekly menu not only helps to save time and money, but also provides a way to create meals with a balance of fat, protein and carbohydrates, plus all of the essential vitamins and minerals needed for the child and adult's body.

Now that we know of the importance of preparation of meals at home, let's move on to talk about meal planning. One of the best ways to make sure that you eat well is to plan your meals ahead of time. It is a vital part of eating a healthy diet, and there are many benefits of meal planning. These benefits include adding variety, eliminating the last minute stress, making shopping easier, saving time and money, helping you to avoid unhealthy choices. Cooking healthy recipes and meals doesn't have to be difficult or time consuming. These healthy recipes will please the whole family. Start your day off with a spring in your step with these simple yet healthy recipes that will keep you energized for the entire day.

But how simple can it be? Well, how about as simple as five minutes of prep time without any cooking needed? Sounds good, doesn't it? Let's dive in no more. Here are eight healthy recipes. Breakfast, fruit cups, papaya boat, tropical eyeopener, chicken TOMMASEO, salad, corn and green chile salad, avocado garden salad, rosemary lemon chicken with vegetables, spaghetti with turkey meat sauce. Let's talk about the breakfast fruit cup all you need or two oranges peeled and seeded and sliced into bite sized pieces. One medium banana peeled and sliced, one tablespoon of raisins, one third cup of low fat vanilla yogurt and one half teaspoon of ground cinnamon. Begin by getting a small bowl and combining the fruit, then divide the fruit equally into four bowls.

Lastly, put a rounded tablespoon of low fat yogurt over fruit in each bowl, then sprinkle on equal amounts of ground cinnamon before serving. The Papy, a boat prepared to papayas, rinsed and peeled one medium banana, peeled and sliced one kiwifruit peeled and sliced into one cup of strawberries about 11 ounces, a can of mandarin oranges drained and three quarter cups of low fat vanilla yogurt, along with one tablespoon of honey and two teaspoons of chopped fresh mint. But that's optional. Now cut the papayas in half lengthwise, scoop out the seeds, place each half in a medium plate, then place an equal amount of banana, kiwifruit, strawberries and oranges in each half of the papaya.

Combine your yogurt, honey and mint and then mix it well and spoon it over the fruit before serving a tropical eyeopener. Prepare your mango peeled and seeded and cut into chunks along with one large banana peeled and sliced, one cup of untrained pineapple chunks and three quarter cups of low fat vanilla frozen yogurt along with one cup of ice cubes. Now combine all of the ingredients in a blender and blend until the mixture is smooth and you can pour into glasses to serve chicken tomato salad. Prepare the dressing with one cup of husk and quartered tomatoes, three tablespoons of light Italian dressing, one fresh Anaheim, Chile seeded and chopped, and one fourth teaspoon of ground black pepper.

As for the salad itself, prepare two cups of chopped cooked chicken or turkey, along with one cup of chopped red bell pepper, one cup of frozen corn thawed and one cup of chopped carrots and slice four green onions and also chop up a quarter cup of cilantro. Now in a blender or a food processor, puree the tomatoes with dressing Anaheim chili and ground black pepper, then set it aside, then combine all of the salad ingredients into a large bowl and toss drizzle the dressing over the salad and toss well to coat, then cover and chill for twenty minutes, or make a day ahead of time to allow flavors to blend and serve on lettuce lined plates or bowls, corn and green chili salad.

All that you need are two cups of frozen corn. Also one 10 ounce can of diced tomatoes with green chilies drained, a half tablespoon of vegetable oil, one tablespoon of lime juice, one quarter cup sliced green onions and two tablespoons of chopped fresh cilantro. Now combine all of the ingredients in a medium bowl, mix well and serve. And now the avocado garden salad. This salad might need a longer prep time, but there's still no cooking needed. Prepare six cups of Toruń or cut mixed salad greens, three medium tomatoes, chopped five green onions, chopped one small cucumber peeled and chopped two tablespoons of lemon juice, one quarter cup teaspoon garlic powder, a half teaspoon of ground black pepper, a half teaspoon of salt and one large avocado peeled. Now mix the salad greens, tomatoes, onions and cucumber in a large serving bowl in a small bowl mix, lemon juice, garlic powder, ground, black pepper and salt.

Pour over the salad mixture and toss it together. Now cut the avocado in half lengthwise, remove the pit and peel the auto cobble halves, then slice into thin wedges about one eighth inch thick, arrange the avocado slices on top of the salad and serve immediately. Rosemary lemon chicken with vegetables. Prepare one half pound of small red potatoes or about three potatoes rinsed and cubed. One and a half cups of baby carrots, one cup of green beans, two trimmed, boneless, skinless chicken breasts halved, which should equal about one pound, one tablespoon of olive oil, one quarter cup of lemon juice, two tablespoons of honey divided, one tablespoon of chopped fresh rosemary or one teaspoon of dried rosemary, along with one teaspoon of grated lemon peel and a quarter cup teaspoon ground black pepper in a medium pot.

Bring eight cups of water to a boil, add the potatoes and carrots and green beans and cook for five minutes, then drain and set to the side, cut the chicken breasts in half place, olive oil and the chicken breasts in a medium skillet and cook over medium for five minutes on each side. Then add your potatoes, carrots, green beans and all of the remaining ingredients to the skillet except for two tablespoons of lemon juice. Cook this over low heat for five minutes or more until the chicken is fully cooked. Then add the remaining lemon juice. To taste and serve spaghetti with turkey meat sauce, you will need a nonstick cooking spray, three quarter pound of lean ground turkey, two cans of diced tomatoes, which should equal to about 14 and a half ounces and juice reserved.

One green bell pepper finely chopped, one cup of finely chopped onion, two cloves of garlic, finely chopped, one teaspoon of dried crushed oregano, one teaspoon of ground black pepper and one pound of spaghetti noodles now spray a large skillet with the nonstick cooking spray, preheat the skillet over medium heat, add the turkey and cook stirring occasionally for five to 10 minutes or until cooked through. Now drain the fat stir in the tomatoes with their juice bell, pepper, onion, garlic and oregano along with the ground black pepper and bring it to a boil and reduce heat cover and simmer for fifteen minutes stirring occasionally. Meanwhile, cook the spaghetti according to the packaged directions, then drain well and serve the sauce over the spaghetti.

Guidelines To Well-being

In this chapter, we are going to talk about the general guideline to overall well-being before going in depth. We should understand that healthy eating is not about strict dietary limitations, staying unrealistically thin or depriving yourself of the food you love. Rather, it's about feeling awesome, improving your health, stabilizing your mood and having more energy. Do you ever feel overwhelmed by all of the conflicting diet and nutrition advice out there? Well, you're not alone. It seems that for every expert who tells you a certain food is good for you, you'll find another saying exactly the opposite. Quite often, convenient foods are laced with too much sugar, salt and other ingredients which are not considered healthy.

These ingredients can often be hidden. So it's important as a part of your education to learn to read food labels while at the grocery, learn what ingredients to avoid as major components are usually listed first in the food labels. Being educated on what is contained within various types of food will help you weed out much of the unhealthy food you may otherwise end up eating permanently. Improving your eating habits requires a thoughtful approach in which you reflect, replace and reinforce. By following these simple approaches, you can cut through the confusion and learn how to create a varied, healthy and tasty diet that's good for your mind and your body. Reflect on all of your specific eating habits, both good and bad, and your common triggers for unhealthy eating.

Replace your unhealthy eating habits with healthier ones. Reinforce your new healthier eating habits. You should create a list of your eating habits. The simplest way to track what you eat and drink is by setting up your diary in a notebook or downloading a food journal app on your phone. This will help you uncover your eating habits. Keep track of everything that goes into your mouth, including all snacks, drinks, meals and even nibbles of food that you eat while you cook. Don't forget to track your total water intake as well. Tracking how much water you drink will give you insight into whether or not you need to consume more water to help you stay hydrated after you've kept your journal for a few days.

Star or highlight areas where you may think you can make changes. For example, you might notice that you don't drink enough water or you typically skip breakfast. These are great areas where you can make healthy changes, highlight the habits, highlight the habits on your list that may be leading you to overeat. Common eating habits that can lead to weight gain are you eat when you're not hungry, you ignore nutrition advice. You're always cleaning your plate. You eat too fast. You are always eating dessert, going wild. On the weekends, you hang out with unhealthy pals. You habitually use food as therapy, you skip meals or perhaps just breakfast.

Awareness is always the first step to change. So make sure you've identified all of the triggers that caused you to engage in those habits. Identify a few that you'd like to work on improving. First, habitual behaviors are driven by cravings for rewards or avoidance of negative consequences. Don't forget to pat yourself on the back for the things you're doing right. It's important to celebrate, which is just as true in life as it is with habits. We want to continue to do things that make us feel good and because an action needs to be repeated for it to become a habit, it's especially important that you reward yourself each time that you practice your new habit.

For example, if you've chosen to have salad instead of a burger as your dinner, celebrate your progress with the reward. It's time to celebrate. Always remember to reward yourself as you make simple changes that in the end will result in achieving your overall goal. Create a list of cues by reviewing your food diary to become more aware of when and where you're triggered to eat for reasons other than hunger. Note how you're typically feeling at those times. Often a particular emotional state or an environmental cue is what encourages eating for non hunger reasons. The common triggers for eating when you're not hungry include suffering from the clean plate syndrome.

The clock says so before or after a stressful meeting or a situation at work, sitting at home while watching television, opening up the cabinet and seeing your favorite snack, coming home after work and having no idea what's for dinner. You can't say no to food pushers and feeling bored or tired and thinking that food might offer a pick me up. Now let's talk about a four step eating habit. Hack No one. Mark the cues on your list. That you encounter on a daily basis or a weekly basis to now ask yourself these questions for each cue you've marked, three, replace unhealthy eating habits with new, healthier ones for finally reinforce your new eating habits, mark the cues on your list that you encountered on a daily or weekly basis.

For example, attending a birthday party may be a trigger for you to have a cheat day to overeat. So simply have that piece of cake that doesn't fit into your daily food intake goals. Thus, you may want to attend as many birthday parties as possible as a cue for you to overeat. Some cues may be absurd as not going to the gym as a cue to binge, but don't fret upon it. Simply mark them down for now. Now ask yourself these questions for each cue that you've marked. Obviously your answer will be no. And you felt like a pig after you binge. Well, your answer may vary.

Just write them down to have clarity and create the pain and disgust. So you know you must change. So you know that you must change. Ask yourself, how can I avoid this cue or situation after noticing the cues and the pain, your non empowering actions brought upon, you find a way to avoid that situation. This option works best for cues that don't involve another party. For example, you choose a different route to work instead of your usual route to avoid going to McDonald's along the way. Or you drink lots of water when you realize that you're in binge mode or change your work desk that was once facing the vending machine or the coffee machine.

You may also choose another place to study instead of your home kitchen. But there are just some events you can avoid, like birthday parties of someone important or a staff meeting. So what do you do? Ask yourself this question for things that I cannot avoid. What can I do differently to eat healthier? The key here is to plan ahead. And when you ask this question beforehand, your brain will naturally find better alternatives to make sure that you stick to your fitness goals. Maybe it's bringing healthy snacks to work, especially when there are long hours ahead. Track your food and make sure it fits your daily macronutrients and don't overeat. Being food conscious in a party is a good way to control yourself.

Eat lots of veggies before attending a party. Being filled before the party is a good way not to binge replace unhealthy eating habits with newer, healthier ones. Now that you've asked yourself the above questions and have a clear sense of awareness, you simply have to take action to replace your old eating patterns. Perhaps you overeat because you're eating too fast, eat slowly. Perhaps you overeat because of hunger, but due to stress, anxiety, anger or frustrations, replace it with non-leading activities like going for a jog, visiting a friend, reading an uplifting book or talking to your family. You'll definitely feel better and you'll totally forget about your hunger. The key to lasting change is to plan ahead.

So write down your daily, weekly and monthly fitness goals, what your food choices are, your body weight goals and stick to it. Finally, reinforce your new eating habits. Rome is not built in a day and neither is your body and your habits. You need to practice your new eating habit day by day, week by week, to rewire your old eating pattern to a new one. But this is the hardest part because it requires patience. Stick with it, believe that it's all worth it. In the end. Special tips to make this work include having a mastermind group to keep each other accountable, join a community, a challenge group and update your close friends and family about your goals.

Picture yourself eating healthy greens and having those washboard abs vibrant, happy and full of energy. One of the best ways to reinforce these habits and make them ingrained into your subconscious mind is to write out a list of one hundred reasons why you want to be fit or eat healthily. Having 100 reasons is going to pull you towards your goal, creating a gravity that guarantees your success as many burn out after pushing too hard for far too long, thus having one hundred reasons, creates that gravity to pull you and your fitness goals almost effortlessly and your fitness goals almost effortlessly. So there you have it, four step eating habit hacks and all the crucial information that you'll ever need to start eating healthy and live a long, strong, fruitful and fulfilling life.

Healthy Binge-Free Lifestyle

Everyone eats to survive, but the type and quality of the food you eat has a tremendous impact on every aspect of your life, not only your physical and mental health. It's also a major factor in determining a person's life expectancy and whether you're likely to contract a major chronic illness in this age of mass produced, highly processed junk food. With all of the chemicals present in today's food and also the increasing rate of inner emotional crisis in modern society, there's no doubt that more and more people are getting sick. People today get sick not only physically, but also psychologically. More people are suffering from problems such as depression, anxiety, frustration, anger issues and low self-esteem.

They're always looking for ways to escape their problems and fill that void in their hearts. And one of the most common ones is through destructive eating behavior, binge eating. Contrary to popular beliefs, binge eating or overeating is not entirely the result of inner emotional and psychological issues. Reasons such as habits, eating patterns, body image, environmental factors and many others can trigger binge eating. Above all, most people overeat simply because they have the urges to binge. So what's the science behind overeating or binge eating, the dangers that come with it? And how do you put an end to overeating and take control of your health once and for all?

Terrifying Food Facts

In this chapter, we'll talk about the terrifying facts food companies don't want you to know. It's not surprising that people are eating so many of the wrong types of foods these days. After all, who has a huge garden full of organic food and the time to tend to it and then prepare healthy meals? Most people today are caught in the rat race. Our ancestors worked very hard to etch out a living, but their work was more directly related to their food production and living conditions being largely hunters and gatherers. And trading was done using things that they had caught, killed or made, rather than doing work that was unrelated to their basic survival. Our ancestors had little use of low nutrient foods. Few people are now able to be self-sufficient and grow their own food.

The vast majority of people have no choice but rely on big food processors and manufacturers to provide the food they need, especially people living in large cities. Huge advertising campaigns by food manufacturers and distributors have an enormous impact on the foods people consume, a lack of nutritional education, misleading advertising as well as decades of government departments and health advisors recommending the wrong types of foods has caused a huge decline in public health. Many processed food or food products that are commonly available are made of substances that should never be ingested. When you go into a supermarket or a convenience store, you'll find aisles and shelves packed full of food products that claim to be healthy and or help you lose weight.

They all have bright, inviting pictures, often of slim, smiling, healthy young people or wording to suggest that they're delicious and also organic or healthy. These are all created by companies that specialize in promoting products and advertising to get you to buy them. Unfortunately, nutritional education in schools is sadly lacking. Instead, the schools often actively support poor eating habits. This is done by allowing unhealthy foods into school canteens, cafeterias and shops. An example is the public school system in America.

Last year, yet another disastrous decision was made, making it mandatory for all pasta served in schools to be fortified with iron. This is because many children are short of iron, and it was hoped this would address the problem. In fact, the pasta was the problem because it was made from bleached white flour that's high in calories and contains almost no nutrients. There's little difference between eating it and eating several spoons of sugar. The added iron is derived from industrial waste and not in the form the body can readily absorb when eaten and is in fact harmful when this is washed down with soda, fruit juice or flavored milk, all of which contain huge amounts of sugar.

It is understandable why people are putting on a lot of weight in the Western world. Many people, including children, are becoming obese. Another example of how the food manufacturing industry is controlling food in the way we look at our food is gluten sensitivity. This is a new multibillion dollar industry making and promoting gluten free foods. Gluten is only one of many proteins in flour. In fact, it's really a minor problem. The main problem is the chemicals that are used to grow wheat, especially GM wheat and glyphosate.

Little did they know that the foods that are most harmful to children and everyone else are the very foods that most people were raised on. Pediatricians often advise young mothers to feed their babies on infant formulas, but these are sugar, soy and chemical based.

A baby's digestive tract is not equipped to metabolize grains. It does not contain the necessary enzymes to break them down into usable compounds because of the lack of salivary amylase to break down grains in the gut, these undigested grains can cause irritation to the gut lining and disrupt the good bacteria cycle. This is known to lead to grain and other food allergies. Later on, grain consumption can also act as an anti nutrient. These properties can prevent a baby or infant from absorbing nutrients from other food. The body then craves for more food so more sugary food is consumed. As a result, the body tries to turn these empty carbohydrates or sugars into glucose and then into body fat. This can lead to the body becoming conditioned to or demanding more sugar or the development of a sweet tooth mentality.

Signs Of Compulsive Overeating

In this chapter, we'll talk about the signs of binge eating disorder or compulsive overeating bed or binge eating disorder is defined by someone who is a compulsive eater, who overeat or consumes an abnormal amount of food in one seating someone who's unable to stop or limit the amount of food he or she eats. At one time, most binge eaters will have at least two episodes a week of binge eating over a six month period. Binge eating disorder can occur in both men and women. It usually results in excessive weight gain, and this can in turn create or reinforce other compulsive eating disorders as people coping with these disorders often feel some degree of guilt and self disgust. Often people with this disorder also have to cope with depression or anxiety.

With these feelings resulting in an increased desire for food to help cope, creating a vicious cycle. These bad disorders are sometimes associated with biological abnormalities such as genetic mutations or hormonal irregularities that also cause compulsive eating addiction. Bed is often associated with people who have, for whatever reason, developed low self-esteem and find it difficult to deal with personal feelings and emotions. Victims of physical, emotional and sexual abuse are also susceptible to eating disorders such as overeating and binge eating. People who are very conscious about their physical appearance are also one of the high risk groups. When subjected to criticism of their weight or body shape, they can develop eating disorders due to shame or embarrassment.

These are some of the emotional and behavioral signs of a typical person with a binge eating disorder. The feeling or experience of being under stress or anxious about anything that can be relieved by eating the inability to finish or stop eating even when full to the point of being uncomfortable, not being able to control what to eat and when to eat, the need to stockpile food for later and the feeling they need to hide their eating behavior from others. The lack of feelings, sensations or real enjoyment from binge eating when a person never really feels they are satisfied or fully satiated when eating, regardless of how much they eat. Always wanting a little more binge eating disorder is known to be the direct, as well as an indirect cause of many complications and health issues.

Various forms of cancer are a common outcome of overeating because of the overload of toxic compounds released into the body's system, such as ammonia, a byproduct of breaking down protein. The chances of having a miscarriage are significantly increased, with overeating and being overweight, a greater chance of cardiovascular disease and increased risk of coronary disease, an increased risk of a stroke, high blood pressure and high blood sugar level type two diabetes, high cholesterol levels, gastrointestinal problems, gallbladder disease, joint and muscle pain, insomnia and sleep apnea. Hypertension, depression and anxiety in order to maintain or support people who have this condition.

There are three types of therapy used CBT or cognitive behavioral therapy, which helps an individual come to terms with their thoughts and feelings, allowing them to understand how and why they have an eating disorder, ITP, or interpersonal psychotherapy, which helps a person focus on their own individual relationships with others, including their families, friends, peers and associates, so they understand how others see them. This is to help them take a realistic look at themselves and their situation with a view to improving their lives and eating habits BGT or dialectical behavior therapy, which helps an individual to learn new skills and methods of coping with their feelings, stress levels and emotions. Until a person is able to gain the motivation and willpower to help themselves, recovery is very unlikely.

Why You Lack Control Around Food

In this chapter, we'll discuss the reasons you're out of control around food. There are many reasons a person may have an eating disorder, especially overeating. Depression is often associated with overeating. Sometimes overeating can be a result of depression, and other times it can be the other way around whereby a person's depression is caused by their eating disorder. Another complex factor that can influence the development of overeating is a person's genetic or biological makeup. The environment you live in and where you grew up can also play a significant role along with your social situation. It's believed that a person's upbringing and social development when young and the way in which they were taught to deal with their emotions and emotional pain or conflicts can have a significant impact on their eating habits and stress related eating patterns.

Studies show that many people who binge can even experience losing consciousness and severely diminished perception of reality. When someone has a long history of overeating and then they try to restrict their food intake, their bodies, biological response will go into famine mode. In other words, their body prepares itself for a period of being deprived of food as a defense mechanism starts to shut down or slow down most of the normal functions in an effort to conserve energy. It also starts to trigger an array of different hunger sensors or natural craving mechanisms whose purpose is to spur the mind into searching for available food sources.

This is a primeval survival technique left over from a time when food was a very scarce commodity and hard to get a hold of the hunger hormone. Ghrelin is responsible for stimulating our appetite. Our body releases it when our stomach is empty and it stops releasing it when our stomach begins to fill while we eat. There are two psychological factors that are working. Our mind decides when we eat. Although we are now creatures of habit, we once and for most of our history were hunters or hunted and gatherers and did not have a pattern of eating regularly, especially not three times a day. Science has not yet been able to explain how we get hungry or why we decide to start eating.

But it's clear that there are many factors that come together to start the mind working in the process of getting us ready to eat. Although we think we are in control of what we eat, we think that our normal, rational and fully conscious brain is deciding what and when we eat. We're very much influenced by physiological forces that most of us are unaware of. Some of the factors that influence our eating, our particular set of genes, our own hormones, the social cues. We recognize the behavior patterns we've learned from environmental factors, including pollution levels, our circadian rhythm, and the amount of energy we've been using the last time we ate something.

Although it is not scientifically proven, it is believed that there are two reasons we eat or rather why we decide to eat. Either we get the nourishment and energy for our bodily needs or homeostatic eating, or we eat to manage our emotions or basically for pleasure or hedonic eating. For most people, it's a matter of trying to do both. They look for food with a high nutritional value, but at the same time they have to enjoy it. This, in theory, would satisfy both the person's emotional and physical needs, and that is if all of the available food had high nutritional content. But in reality, most of the food that is easily available to everyone today is highly processed food or junk food.

These types of food are almost always made with a very low nutritional content, but a very high carbohydrate and chemical content. So it tastes good, highly addictive, but destroys your body. Burning question that no one wants to address is why people actually want to eat so much and why it's so hard for them to stop. This is not a question of willpower, although some people with exceptionally strong willpower, although they are unlikely to be overeaters, will probably find it not so difficult to stop overeating.

For most of us, the answer highly depends on our body types, how it reacts around food, our metabolism rate and natural eating patterns. Our body evolved in a hunter gatherer mode. It was not designed to eat the three square meals a day many health and nutritional advisors have been trying to convince us of for decades. Our natural feeding rhythm is probably more like all other mammals in the world. They eat when they find or catch their food and have a cycle of eating.

What's available and storing any excess that they have consumed is fat. Then waiting for the next meal while waiting or sleeping, they would have been relying on using up their fat reserves. A natural feast and famine cycle. Eating is often done on autopilot and our conscious mind hardly notices it. Have you experienced instances? When you snack on a bag of chips while doing something else, such as watching television but don't remember doing so until the whole bag is empty, this is an example of your over-eating habits, taking over your actions and subconscious mind without you knowing it.

The Dangers Of Overeating

In this chapter, we'll talk about the dangers of overeating, the danger of overeating, apart from the obvious fact that you'll get fat. Is that the foods that people tend to overeat are usually unhealthy. They are largely made up of empty carbohydrates that wouldn't trigger the body's built in safeguards to stop you from overeating. With the majority of people living not far from supermarkets and fast food restaurants, there's little chance that most people will go hungry. The big challenge is to find healthy and inexpensive foods. When you overeat, it's most likely to be the unhealthiest food. Think about it. Hardly anyone will overeat or binge feed on bean sprouts or broccoli shoots, winter greens or cauliflower.

However, sugar and carbohydrates are not the only culprits to overeat. Oftentimes people tend to overeat meat proteins, which will burden your entire body system, especially your kidneys. The human body is a very complex system that has evolved countless times to protect itself from both internal and external threats. One of these defense systems is cancer protection. Our pancreas produces an enzyme called trips, and this enzyme has a specific function in our body that is to break down the protective protein covering those defective mutant cells in our bodies. These mutant cells are the only cells that have this type of protection.

It stops the white blood cells or immune system from being able to destroy them. When we consume too much meat protein, we use up our supply of chips in allowing mutant or cancerous cells to multiply. This is because the secondary job of trips is to break down meat protein. It should be noted that protein from plants does not have this effect as our bodies do not need trips and to break down vegetable proteins. The average person needs to consume about 35 grams of protein each meal to cater for all the normal internal bodily functions and replace worn muscles, etc..

When we consume more than thirty five grams of protein, this extra protein will be broken down into sugars with the main byproducts of ammonia and uric acid going into the bloodstream. Uric acid is the main cause of gout, a very painful arthritic condition that affects a lot of people. The ammonia is responsible for premature aging. It can cause headaches, harms many internal organs, and is suspected of being a catalyst for many types of cancer. Our immune system suffers when we overeat foods that are high in sugar.

This includes all processed flour products such as bread, pastries, pasta, most confectionery and a whole host of other mainly processed foods containing empty carbohydrates. A typical dessert, such as a banana split, contains as much as 24 teaspoons of refined or table sugar. There are about eight and a half teaspoons of refined table sugar in a Snickers bar, and a 12 ounce bottle of Coke has about nine teaspoons of refined table sugar. A person's immune system will become paralyzed and unable to function for about four to six hours.

If that person consumes 25 teaspoons of refined or table sugar, it's due to the effect it has on the white blood cells. This condition leaves a person exposed to all manner of infection and destroys the body's natural cancer protection. The short term effects of overeating often includes a feeling of being lethargic and feeling bloated. This is a temporary condition for those who occasionally overeat and is not considered a major health threat. But there are serious health implications for people who habitually overeat or are chronic overeaters. This is because they cause their entire system at all levels to become stressed and inflamed, which is now believed to be a leading or major cause of most of today's chronic medical conditions.

Most people are not aware that the average person needs about 1500 to 2000 calories each day. Approximately 1000 of those are used to keep your body going on essential activities. The other 800 calories are used to provide daily activities such as moving and the energy for those daily activities. When you exceed the number of calories you need by overeating, your body stores the extra calories as body fat and your weight increases. If you take careful measurements of your weight, you can see over a period of, say, a week if you are losing, gaining or maintaining a steady weight, this is a good indication of whether you are overeating or not. One pound of body weight is equal to thirty five hundred calories.

So to gain one pound of body weight, you need to consume an extra 3500 calories. And to lose one pound of body weight, you need to reduce your intake by five hundred or burn up an extra 500 calories every day for a week. If the food you mainly overeat are cooked in low quality fats such as vegetable oils, or you mainly eat high carbohydrate and sugary foods, you can get what is known as a sugar rush. The sugar rush results in a high spike in your blood sugar levels, which puts a huge strain on all your internal organs. You will experience a short term surge in energy levels. You might even experience a crash feeling fatigue and sluggish after the surge.

These types of foods can cause a variety of digestive issues, including bloating and excess. Being overweight has complications for your heart and also your joints and ligaments, these can become worn and stressed because when someone is overweight or obese, there's a lot of additional weight or pressure placed on the body. Someone who constantly overeats is likely to become overweight, even if they're reasonably active. This extra body weight volume can affect a person's self-esteem or self-image in a negative way. The more you eat, the more weight you gain and the less confident a person feels about themselves.

It's been shown that this can lead to depression, anxiety issues, intimacy and sexual difficulties, as well as antisocial behavior and an unusual and unnatural attitude to food and eating in general. It's expected that when a person is able to take control of their eating habits and stop overeating, many of these problems will naturally be resolved upon loss of excess weight so a person can have a much better self-image and improved mental health.

The 10 Types Of Overeating

In this chapter, we'll learn about the 10 types of overeating. There are many different reasons people overeat. It's not as straightforward as the idea that fat people are just being greedy. In fact, as we've already covered, for many people, the compulsion to overeat is very hard to control. Overeating can lead to heartburn, discomfort and stomach pain in the short term, as well as gastrointestinal problems, flatulence, bloating and diarrhea, heart problems, cancers and obesity. In the long term, most people who normally do not overeat can find doing so quite unpleasant and uncomfortable. But those who frequently overeat find that their body release is a natural pleasure chemical to adjust for excessive food intake, making it actually enjoyable to overeat or at least encourage us to feel like continuing to want to consume more.

This is the start to forming a type of food addiction. The following are examples of overeating, one consuming large amounts of food, much more than a normal person would at one time. And doing so quickly is considered binge eating. A single or occasional act of binge eating is not necessarily harmful in itself. But if you have a habit of eating this way, it's considered a symptom that can lead to an eating disorder or bulimia nervosa. Ordering and consuming supersize meal portions is another sign of overeating. There are now a large number of establishments who offer all you can eat and very large or super sized portions.

These meals are usually made with low cost and low quality ingredients. So although you're getting a large volume of food, you're actually getting very little nourishment, which causes your body to seek more food to compensate. All this excess food is usually in the form of empty carbohydrates and turned into body fat. The normal cycle of using the food you consume for powering and repairing your body with any extra being turned into fat and then used as needed stops. Instead of burning the stored fat, your body just burns. A portion of the carbohydrates you consume in any excess just goes into your body's fat stockpile in a never ending cycle.

So you get bigger and unhealthier. Three, because the body has developed a series of senses that stimulates the brain with chemical messages when triggered, a person learns to use these triggers to make themselves feel better when they are under some type of emotional stress or strain. This is acceptable occasionally. But when a person is prone to emotional mood swings, depression, or they often have feelings of being unhappy, upset or sad, they can find they have an emotional overeating problem. This is because they are using food triggers to make themselves feel better with the result of overeating or binge eating for an overeating disorder very similar to emotional overeating, disorder can happen to those who are suffering from stress.

This can cause people to feel anxious instead of depressed. This type of over eating disorders are often associated with people who have a heavy workload or work long hours without taking time off for adequate rest and meals. When you eat rapidly, especially when you're on the run, there's a high tendency to overeat or binge. The simple explanation for this is because the stomach does not have time to relay the full signals to the brain, which normally stops a person from eating when he's full. Five sugar type food addictions are a major cause of overeating.

Often they form at a very young age, usually starting when babies and children are given foods, high sugar content. Not only do people who crave sugar often become overweight, they are more likely to have dental problems and high blood sugar levels. These factors will lead to diabetes. Studies suggest that a high sugar diet is a major cause of emotional issues. A trap many people fall into is having a healthy, wholesome meal, then following it with a sugar laden dessert or drinks that negate many of the benefits they would have had from their meal. Instead of using sugar, think about using spices such as cinnamon to sweeten your food or drinks. Cinnamon helps to slow your food as it travels through your digestive system.

Give your food a new dimension by adding a small amount of cider vinegar as it improves flavor and helps lower the food glycemic index. So like with cinnamon, you metabolize food at a slower rate. Six. If you feel hungry, try drinking water. Oftentimes people mistake hunger with thirst. Seven snacking on junk foods between meals is partially difficult, snacking on junk foods between meals is a partially difficult thing to stop for many people and can lead to overeating. If you feel the need to snack, pick snack foods that are healthy and nourishing, such as vegetables, like carrots, celery or salads, fruit and nuts are also wholesome food choices.

But the total calorie count for the day should be taken into account if you're trying to reduce your bodyweight or daily calories intake. Eight many people now get a substantial part of their weekly food diet from fast foods, this makes eating normal volumes of food very difficult because fast foods are purposely designed to make you want to eat more of them. They have in their ingredients carefully formulated chemical additives to make them react with your taste buds, sending messages to your brain that the body needs more of this. Furthermore, these compounds are highly addictive, coupled with their very low nutrient content and huge amount of high calorie carbohydrates, as well as refined salts and oils. These foods are catalysts to make you overeat and result in obesity.

Nine A lot of good people fall into the trap of finding comfort in eating food. Sometimes this can be a good thing as long as you are careful about selecting the right types of foods and balance your eating with a reasonable amount of physical activity. Another major lifestyle issue most people have today is that they always pick the wrong food and don't exercise. Even worse, they incorporate eating as a means of coping with their emotions. There are people who indulge in food when they're happy, sad, frustrated, stressed, angry and all different emotions. They become dependent on food as a remedy for their own self comfort. 10 social eating can also lead to another type of over eating disorder.

Oftentimes, social eating involves consuming large amounts of food and drinks spread over a relatively long period. Attending these social events occasionally is not a problem. Those who often eat socially can feel they are obliged to eat and possibly drink more than they normally would often. These meals are high in calories and not very filling, so people tend to consume them in large volumes. 11. Some people find that they are at a loose end or do not have enough things to occupy their minds. They become bored. So in place of other stimulation, they resort to eating just to relieve themselves from boredom. These people are most likely to become binge eaters and go for supersize portions like fast foods, as well as taking part in excessive snacking of predominantly junk foods.

Great Strategies To Prevent Overeating

In this chapter, we'll talk about strategies to prevent overeating, the compassionate mind approach to beating overeating. Everyone's aware of the fact that obesity rates are getting higher each year, despite the many millions of dollars pumped into health care each year in the US. Americans now eat an average of three thousand seven hundred seventy five calories a day. That's one thousand seven hundred seventy five more than what they need. When you consume more calories than your body really needs, it will be stored as extra energy known as fats, with people consuming almost twice as much as they need consistently.

The population in general can only get fatter. The old saying information is power is also true for information on eating habits. And if you know what is happening with the food you choose to eat and how your body reacts to it and different foods you are on the way to being able to beat the problem of overeating. Once you have an understanding of how your metabolism works and how many calories you actually need to sustain your daily activities, then it's possible to make meal plans and menus that are designed to meet both your physical and emotional needs.

A diet that is bland and boring, which is non filling and provides no pleasure from eating, is doomed to failure. Making a menu that is tailored to your own unique preferences is the best option. The first thing you should attempt to do in order to stop overeating is to start cutting back a little at a time. If you have the habit of drinking three cans of soda a day, try cutting down to one. This will save you from consuming 300 calories a day. Think about making, not buying ready made musingly for breakfast. A half cup contains one hundred and fifty calories and provides a huge array of useful nutrients to make it interesting. A more palatable Servet with organic cream or coconut cream, about fifty calories per tablespoon and some fresh fruit.

This will provide you a filling and tasty breakfast that will keep you feeling full until lunchtime and you will not feel the need for snacking. A high protein breakfast suits many people and is likely to set you up well for the day and lessen the likelihood of binge eating during lunch or dinner time. By taking control of your diet and eating habits, you can have less desire to overeat. Carving out a diet or meal plan is a good start. Try planning out your whole week's meal plan or menus. Here's a tip for you. And planning out your meals. Choose foods that complement each other, contain high natural fiber and nutrients, and low in carbs or sugars to ensure that you'll feel full and nourished after meals.

Foods such as vegetables, nuts, beans and legumes can reduce your tendency to overeat. But don't forget to keep things interesting and make sure that your meal plans are giving you the feeling of satiety most of the time. Then reward yourself once a week with an activity you enjoy so that you stop binging or overeating before it becomes a habit. A lot of condiments are very high end sugar and other natural compounds. Tomato sauce, which is the undisputed favorite source worldwide, is a prime example in a teaspoon of commercial tomato sauce. There are twenty calories in homemade tomato sauce. There are only five calories. So why the 15 calorie difference? Commercial sauce tends to have more sugar and processed ingredients in it to make it more flavorful and addictive.

But at the same time it destroys your health in the long run. Fifteen calories may look little, but this number adds up over time. So why not create your own healthy source? The ingredients are easy to find and don't require much effort to create. Basically, anyone can prepare it at home. Here's a healthy recipe for tomato sauce. Place two pounds of tomatoes, a mixture of acid free and beef tomatoes, half pound appended diced pumpkin and chopped onion, foreclosure of garlic, a few peppercorns, several Baileys and a few cloves. Place it all together in a pressure cooker for thirty minutes, a stockpot for two hours or a crock pot for eight hours. Add salt to taste at the end of the cooking time. Tomato mush will be formed next. Pass this through a fine mesh strainer to remove any solids and the sauce will be ready to serve.

You can also prepare the sauce in thicker consistency as desired and finally keep it refrigerated for a week. For the best result. This sauce tastes great with some herbs, capsicum, chili, ginger and others. As a finishing touch. You can use it on everything and anywhere else tomato sauce goes. Not only will it save you a lot of money, it will help you reduce your calorie count and liven up many dishes without ingesting too much sugar. When the stomach is empty, it has a high volume of about one and a half ounces. But when it's full, a normal stomach can expand to between a quarter and one gallon. It's part of nature's design to have a stomach that stretches with that stretching monitor. Your brain knows how much it's stretching.

Your body will send signals to the brain, letting it know how much food is coming through. Some messages are chemical and others travel via nerves, such as the vagus nerve that goes from your abdomen to your head. While you're eating different hormones, send different messages. Colliss to Kynan is released by the gut. When we consume protein and fat, this chemical informs the brain to stop eating other foods. Hormones are released to slow down the passage of food through the system or to stop. Any more food from entering insulin is also released to deal with carbohydrates and excess proteins as both are turned into sugar or glucose, the body's primary energy source, when it does not have fats to burn.

The interesting thing is that many of these hormones stay in the system and can affect the next meal. This is only true unless there's too much empty carbohydrates and unnatural chemicals like junk foods overrunning these delicate systems. It's totally fine to indulge in occasional treats, such as having a once a week cheap meal without going overboard. What really matters is to make sure that you're constantly maintaining your ideal weight in optimum health. This can only be done if you're consistent in executing a long term strategy to overcome overeating and binge eating. Although even an occasional feast or treat is OK, it's essential to keep your body, especially your digestive system, working efficiently day after day.

The long term nutrient and energy needs of our body are catered by the leptin feedback loop. This helps the brain make decisions on how much food and what type of the different nutrients need to be absorbed from the food being metabolized. The necessary calorie intake, the use of energy where it's taken from and where any excess needs to be stored are also dealt with by this loop. This is all decided by the brain from the information sent by the hormone leptin that is released by the body's fat tissue. Leptin tells the brain how much energy is stored as body fats and how much energy we're consuming at any moment.

The level of leptin in the blood is directly related to our body fat. The more fat we have, the more leptin circulates in our system. This feedback loop is important as it functions as a natural mechanism to maintain the balance of our body weight and energy level. The decisions made by the brain are based on leptin levels, which are themselves then adjusted by the brain to optimum levels. Completing the loop. Our leptin feedback loop is like many systems in our body. It was developed by evolution to suit all the natural conditions the human body could encounter.

Leptin works perfectly for those who consume a largely wholesome, mainly organic diet. On the other hand, it can't cope with some of the highly processed, low nutrient foods that many people consume regularly. In fact, it often just stops working when it encounters salty, sweet, creamy chemical foods with virtually no nutrients. Although they give our senses a wonderful workout and taste delicious, they really should be avoided. If you want to stop overeating and obtain your ideal weight, having these types of diets well over the long term makes us leptin resistant and inflames the brain. They usually cause a person to feel less satisfied and needing to eat more.

The junk food industry is a master of getting people addicted to their foods filled with chemicals and additives. These foods are engineered to be super palatable, a term that describes the whole experience of eating and the pleasure that we get from food palatability is probably the thing that influences the amount of food we eat at each meal. These foods are engineered to taste so good that you cannot resist them. Once you munch on them, it'll trigger your cravings and you'll have a hard time resisting these foods. From then onwards, when these two sensations or tastes are put together, you create a mixture that for many is irresistible.

They just have to have it again and again. Basically, it becomes an instant addiction for many that destroys their health, but also a highly profitable combination for the junk food manufacturers. It's a sad trap for many people as these foods are purposely engineered for people to always binge on them. Sometimes they even go to extraordinary lengths for junk food. Oftentimes those who try these foods once will have them for a second or even third time. Just like any other addictions, people can lose self-control when they're addicted to junk food. These are some of the nasty combinations that result in binge eating foods that are high density.

High energy equals lots of calories in a very small packet, foods with a very high fat content, foods made from highly refined starch, foods made from highly refined sugars, foods filled with artificial sweeteners, foods filled with lots of refined salt, foods that have a special texture like crunchy or creamy foods containing drugs like alcohol or caffeine, foods with high amounts of flavor enhancers like MSG. Ninety nine percent of the food combinations mentioned earlier cannot be found in nature. But our man made it creates a brain versus body situation where our brain tells us to eat more and binge, whereas our body rejects these types of food. As a result, more and more people are suffering from multiple health diseases today than ever before.

Overcoming An Overeating Disorder

In this chapter, we'll learn how to overcome an eating disorder, this is a hotly debated topic by many health professionals. Some claim that overeating is a real addiction and others claim there's no factual basis for calling overeating or binge eating an addiction. It's obvious that overeating causes many health issues, but many suggest that this is a symptom of some much more serious illness. They believe that getting to the root of the illness is the only real treatment. Sadly, many people don't consider binge eating a problem until they're obese or severely ill. They considered that food addiction is only a problem when it's harmful to someone else.

Most government departments are now trying to educate the people. Many schools are beginning to introduce programs to educate students about the benefits of exercising regularly and practicing a healthy, wholesome diet. In order to overcome binge eating, you must first make a conscious decision that you want to change. After that, you need to put in place a strategy that will help you accomplish your goals of not overeating and presumably losing weight or at least gaining your optimum weight and overall health. The following are some useful strategies to control what you eat. Think of your body as a complete and working system, a living machine. It needs to be looked after and stay balanced.

The food you eat today can and will affect you physically and mentally tomorrow or any day in the future. What you ate last night affects what you and your body feel this morning, as your breakfast will affect your performance throughout the entire day. Try to consume less processed food and, if possible, consume more organic, fresh products. If your diet consists of mainly unprocessed food, you'll have a hard time over eating. As these foods are more substantial and filling, they also take much longer time to digest. So you won't easily feel hungry. Base your diet around home, preferably fresh or minimally cooked foods that you enjoy eating.

Remember that even though some whole fresh organic foods are much more expensive than standard processed foods, they contain a lot more nutrients. So in reality, choosing fresh organic foods are far more cost effective as you're getting more quality over quantity. Eat enough high quality protein as when you eat protein, it is more satisfying and you tend to eat fewer calories overall than if you mainly eat carbohydrates. Try to eat about thirty five grams of protein each meal. Fresh vegetables or frozen organic vegetables, especially those with natural bright colors, are known to be super foods. Try to include as many vegetables into your diet as possible.

They are low in calories and high in essential nutrients, perfect to curb craving and keep you full and healthy at all times. Try to get your carbohydrates or starchy vegetables such as tubers like potatoes, sweet potato, cassava, yam and carrots. Parsnips, turnips and beets. Beans and legumes are a good source, as is fruit, because you get a good amount of fiber and roughage as well as many essential nutrients combined with them. These foods take a longer time to digest and stay in your system longer. Therefore, your internal satiety sensors will tell your brain that you're not hungry so there's no need for snacks or binge eating. The human body burns carbohydrates, alcohol, protein and fat for fuel.

But carbohydrates are not essential for survival. In fact, you can live without any. The main advantage of carbohydrates is they provide relatively quick energy. The main fuel for the body is glucose, a form of sugar. And this is essential for brain function and powering your body. Our bodies turn carbohydrates, protein, fat and alcohol into glucose, always starting with the one that is easiest to convert to energy, which is usually carbohydrates. If there's no carbohydrate, first use alcohol and fat for energy, then protein. Fat is arguably the best fuel to use to give energy to your body as long as you choose. Only good quality fats do not use any refined vegetable oils at all, including margarines or vegetable shortening or lard.

They are not healthy. Use only refined coconut, palm and olive oils and butter or lard from free range organic livestock. Or get your fat and oil from fresh avocado, olives, nuts, ocean caught fish or by eating pasture raised organic free range livestock. Taking your time eating and chewing your food is very important. It gives your system time to adjust to the arrival of the new food and for your brain to monitor its effect, taking the little extra time it takes to make your meals exciting and appetizing, and then savoring each bite, sensing the flavor, texture and aroma and enjoying each mouthful is a very healthy and sensible approach to eating. Many people shoving as much as possible, as fast as possible into their mouths. Much of it gets swallowed without being properly chewed.

And the. Result is that any nutrients it contains are able to pass through the system without being absorbed. This is mainly due to the fact that many processed foods are already in a state where when you put them in your mouth, they feel like they're already chewed. This is nothing you can really sink your teeth into, like a good piece of steak and a healthy salad. An excellent approach to stopping yourself from overeating is to use smaller plates with smaller portions and eat your meal slowly making a dinner or a meal up of many different small dishes or Books, and using the meal as the main entertainment with pleasant table talk and enjoying the company of others was the accepted way of dining in many places several hundred years ago, often with the extended family included.

With today's habits of eating in front of the TV or driving through fast food restaurants, it's becoming very hard to sit down and enjoy a meal. A good strategy is to make it inconvenient to get a hold of fast or processed foods. Don't keep them in your refrigerator or pantry. If you really want them, then make it so you have to go out to get them. Take a special trip just to buy junk foods that maybe you will not bother so often and settle for a healthy alternative. One of the biggest mistakes many people make is to stop eating all the things they enjoy at once or going cold turkey. That's OK if you can, but it should be recognized that it's also OK to allow yourself on occasion to have the food you really like.

But no are bad for you. Just treat them in the same way as your other food, eat them mindfully or slowly and enjoy the taste and sensation you've been craving. Enjoy savoring them to the last bit without any guilt. Just accept that sometimes you deserve a treat. After that you can try harder and achieve new milestones. If you wish to put an end to overeating and binge eating, you should first leverage your effort by determining what is your outcome, how much do you wish to weigh? What's the purpose of doing so? It can be for your health, fitness and vitality, or it can be for your family and loved ones and finally figuring out how you're going to achieve it. One surefire way to rewire your brain is to think about how you feel towards eating.

Ask yourself, do you think of food all the time? Is it something that consumes you or are you content until something alerts you to a food or snack? How do you feel before you eat? What do you feel while you are eating? How do you feel after eating? Are you always hungry no matter how much you eat? Do you eat because you feel hungry or do you eat because you think you should? Or just because it's a habit at lunch or dinner time? Do you crave certain foods, candy or chocolates? How about thinking about a fresh, ripe mango, strawberry or apricot instead? Do you think this would be a good alternative? Think about making your own healthy chocolate using Cacao or organic butter and raw honey or maple syrup.

Would this appeal to you? How often do you feel hungry after each meal? Are you a fast eater or a slow eater? Are you angry about your eating habits? Do you get impatient or bad tempered if you have to wait for food? The whole idea is to get you thinking about why you are hungry. Why is it necessary for you to eat right now? With today's busy lifestyles, many people tend to forget about the pleasure they can get from mindful eating. In some countries like France and Italy, mindful eating is considered the norm, the cornerstone of these cultures. It's interesting that although France holds the record for the highest dairy fat consumption of any Western country, the people don't find it necessary to diet to the same degree as most other countries.

As there are a lot fewer illnesses associated with the diet, America has over twice the amount of people that have weight problems as Italy and France. A new approach to overcome binge eating and overeating is to avoid having huge meals and consume lots of small, high quality meals. So you never feel hungry. If you select the right foods to snack on, you'll be able to eat less easily. Also, you won't have to experience the usual cycle of feeling full of energy and then being tired later on as you'll have a steady stream of energy throughout the day.

Final Ideas & Tips

That brings us to the end of this chapter, Of course. I hope it has helped you understand what overeating is all about and gives you some ideas on different ways you can go about developing new healthy eating platforms. Eating can and should be one of life's greatest pleasures from growing or finding your food to preparing it, cooking it, and finally savoring the fruits of your labors rather than just rushing into a fast food place and grabbing whatever to devour. I sincerely hope that you found this chapter Book useful. I wish you all the best in this journey towards developing new healthy eating patterns. Thank you and good luck.

Proven Steps And Strategies

This chapter, Of course, contains proven steps and strategies on how to begin your own vegan diet, how to maintain and acquire the type of body you wish on a vegan diet and presents to you athletes and prominent individuals who debunk some of the greatest myths when it comes to the world of vegan eating. Many individuals believe that a vegan lifestyle is not a lifestyle conducive to muscle building or psychological health. Many believe vegans cannot possibly obtain the protein sources they need in order to keep their bodies working efficiently. And others believe that a vegan lifestyle is not one that should be held for the long haul.

Many people are under the assumption that in order to live a healthy and productive life inside and outside of the gym, one has to constantly chug protein shakes and energy supplements in order to improve performance. Well, we are here to let you know that none of these are true. This chapter Book will have real life athletes who not only live a vegan lifestyle, but prove that performance and muscle building are not simply based on the idea of laboratory manufactured and animal based protein sources. This chapter, Of course, will talk about the true dietary needs of vegans and where they get their sauces from, and it will compare to the types of nutrients and proteins other dietary lifestyles obtain in order to show that vegans do not simply go without.

They just choose to broaden their food based horizons. Not only that, but many people believe that a vegan lifestyle cannot possibly give someone the energy they need in order to go workout in a gym for two hours. Well, not only will this be yet another myth debunked within the Book, but it will also be something we address in full. That is, we will outline various workout plans and routines that will benefit the vegan lifestyle you have chosen or are at least curious about in order to achieve the physical benefits you want for your own body.

Yes, it is possible to build muscle on a vegan diet and yes, it is possible to keep up these cardio based marathons on a vegan diet. In fact, you'll be genuinely surprised as to how similar the workout routines are of those who eat vegan and those who do not. Vegans are not individuals who shove their beliefs down someone's throat. They're individuals who are merely passionate about abstaining from the use of animal products. They do not consume them. And in some individuals, they even attempt to not use them. Are they extremists? Yes, but there are extremists in every healthy lifestyle. This chapter Book contains dietary outlines for those who are or want to be vegan.

Exercise guidelines for those eating this type of food, lifestyle and athletes that will be highlighted in order to show real life examples as to how this works. Not only that, but these athletes will have their own personal testimonies as to why they began this lifestyle and how it has benefited them in the long run. And if that was not enough, all of those dreaded myths perpetuated about the vegan lifestyle will finally be debunked. Welcome to the new and amazing world of vegan warriors.

The Vegan Journey - Health & Vitality

In this chapter, we'll talk about the vegan journey for health and performance. Living a vegan lifestyle has many different benefits. Backed up by multiple prominent research studies, it has been proven that a vegan lifestyle can lower the risk of cardiac events, reduce the risk of developing certain cancers and lower an individual's chance of Type two diabetes. Not only that, but it helps with regulating one's metabolism and weight and can stave off certain weight induced phenomena such as hypertension. A vegan lifestyle has also proven to reduce someone's risk of stroke. But there are many different benefits to a vegan lifestyle that are not merely based on health.

The UN recently released a report that stated a dire need for the world to migrate away from consistently consuming animal products. The impact from a majority of the world's growing population, consuming meat and animal products is the growing need for crops to feed those animals in order to breed them for food. Food is not like finding an alternative for fossil fuels. People are required to eat for their survival. However, as the current population stands, animals raised for the sole purpose of providing food to the general population consume over half of all the world's crops. Yes, half. And no, that is not some random statistic. That statistic was embedded within the UN's official report.

It is simply an inefficient use of our planet's natural resources. As the population continues to grow because of the advancement in medicine, more agricultural space is going to be necessary in order to grow and feed the highest number of animals bred necessary for food purposes. Many people talk about deforestation and scream for it to go away. But many people do not understand that around 56 percent of that deforestation is going to the purpose of agriculture. Growing food not simply for humans, but for those animals that are raised specifically for general food sources. And if that's not enough, around eight hundred and fifty million people, around 15 percent of the entire world's population, struggle and deal with undernourishment.

Even with all of this going on, it's almost simply a waste of the planet's natural resources that will become exhausted in the near future if we continue on this path. So what does being vegan have to do with any of this? Well, not consuming animal products and meat takes a bit off the burden of this need for more agricultural space for those animals we need to feed. Adopting a vegan lifestyle takes the stress off the planet's natural resources and will ultimately require less water, fossil fuels and land in order to cultivate. Multiple reports have surfaced that declare the world's population will be around nine billion individuals by 2050, and many more studies have been done that proclaim the world's meat needs will not be sustainable.

By that point, adopting a vegan lifestyle can help that statistic. Many vegans scream about animal cruelty and how that should be the reason everyone converts to a vegan lifestyle. But the truth is more that people are concerned about their own well-being rather than the well-being of an animal they cannot see, touch or hear. So it should bring a smile to many people's faces when we say that there are more scientifically backed studies that give even more personal health benefits that are only provided when adopting a vegan diet. It's been shown in various studies that a vegan diet provides a higher availability of fiber, potassium, antioxidants and folate, which makes it the most mineral and vitamin rich diet offered on the health and wellness circuit today. Not only that, but it's the number one recommended diet by general physicians and specialists when it comes to someone who needs to lose weight.

One particularly renowned study compared a vegan diet to a dozen other popular and well received diets and found that the participants who adopted the vegan diet lost the most weight, with an average of nine point three pounds more than all the other groups of participants utilizing other diets. It can also help level out blood sugar levels and promote kidney functions as a result of lowering and regulating internal blood sugars. Not only that, but it has been proven to help individuals who suffer with different arthritic pains because many of the vegetables and fruits ingested contain antioxidants and free radicals. Yes.

Those are actually a thing that help manage internal swelling, however, no one can deny the social stigma and misconceptions many people have because of the loud and proud vegans who accuse people of being monsters because they eat meat. Unfortunately, they are out there with any lifestyle, whether it be health based, politically based or religiously based. Those who take it to an extreme and give the lifestyle a bad reputation. Luckily, there are ways you can combat that social stigma should you choose to adopt a vegan diet and or lifestyle. For starters, educate yourself, look into those studies and hold those statistics at the ready.

With taboo subjects come people who will want you to prove to them what you are talking about. So be ready, read and educate yourself in the avenues that have proven a vegan lifestyle does what it claims to do. Many other people believe vegans are not getting what they need when it comes to macro and micronutrients. Take, for example, proteins and calcium. Once someone hears someone does not eat meat or animal byproducts, they automatically assume two things are not being ingested: calcium from milk and protein from meat. This is another avenue to properly educate someone.

Use your thirst for knowledge and research foods that are rich in calcium and protein that are not stereotypical resources. Not only should you incorporate those into your diet, you can also use this information when educating someone on what veganism really is versus what they have been originally introduced to. Another way to get around this social stigma, if you've not educated yourself fully yet, is to simply say you enjoy the taste of something while not enjoying the taste of something else. If you go out to a restaurant and order a vegan based dish, someone will eventually ask If you aren't vegetarian, why are you eating a vegetarian dish instead of telling them? Because I'm a vegan and spiraling into that social stigma conversation.

Rephrase what you would say to them. Instead, tell them because you thought the dish would taste good or because you enjoy the taste of fried tofu versus the fried chicken they were offering. No one can argue with you if it's simply a matter of what your taste buds in your stomach prefer at the moment. But someone will always argue with you over ideologies. However, education on the diet and lifestyle will be necessary at some point in time, especially if you ever want to talk about your eating habits with someone. Luckily, we have many different popular myths in the next chapter that are easily and scientifically debunked to help begin your mental journey towards preparing for all aspects of your lifestyle, including the diet.

Debunking Vegan Myths

In this chapter, we'll talk about debunking the myths. There are many different myths about the vegan community that perpetuate society, some of them are large myths that have spread to the far corners of the world, and some of them are lesser known myths that could wreak havoc on the community if believed by the general public. We're here to introduce you to these myths right before we debunk them completely. Myth number one, vegans don't get enough protein in their diets. This is simply false. While meat and things like eggs and milk are major sources of protein, they are not the only ones. Many of our beloved vegetables have protein like spinach.

One cup of uncooked spinach has around seven grams of protein. Nut butter has eight grams of protein per two tablespoons. Quinoa has around nine grams of protein per cooked cup and one cup of cooked lentils packs a whopping 18 grams of protein. Many research studies have shown, in fact, that both vegans and traditional eaters are usually getting too much protein in their diets. Myth number two, if you can't eat meat, then you can't build muscle to become strong. There is so much false in this statement. It's unbelievable. Things like hemp powder and dairy deprived whey protein sources pack incredible volumes of protein, just like those traditional protein shakes that are beloved to bodybuilders.

And the foods listed previously are perfect meat protein replacements when it comes to taking in the required amount of protein in order to build and keep muscles strong. However, another myth also flows into this point as well. It is possible to get the recommended amount of calcium into a vegan diet without drinking and eating dairy products that will enable someone to keep muscles and bones healthy for the long term. Things like raw nuts, calcium fortified hemp milk and cooked greens like broccoli and kale have great amounts of calcium in them per serving. Myth number three, vegans are weak.

First off, what? Secondly, no NFL defensive lineman David Carter, a six time Ironman champion John Joseph and the tennis sisters Venus and Serena Williams are all vegans. Need I say more? Myth number four. Vegan diets are not healthy. If fruits, vegetables, non GMO products, no MSG and lack of meat and dairy are somehow unhealthy, then you've got me here. However, I highly doubt a diet that comes recommended by oncologists for certain cancer patients is unhealthy. Not only does a vegan lifestyle afford the body more opportunities to acquire micro and macro nutrients, the body needs to operate and survive. It also helps to flush out the toxins and free radicals that have built up within the body that have been deposited by overprocessed foods, grain fed, animal meats and even over pasteurized dairy products.

Myth number five, you will have to supplement holes in your diet with vitamins if you go vegan, which will end up costing you more money. All right, let's break this one down. Supplements for holes in the diet. A vegan diet has been scientifically researched and measured against dozens of other diets. And it's come out on top time and time again as the most nutrient dense diet on the planet. The only reason people who attempt a vegan eating lifestyle end up having to supplement with vitamins is because simply cutting out animal products and dairy is only half the battle. The other part is then replacing those things you've removed with things.

You can then ingest the idea of supplements costing you money, which makes a vegan diet somehow unattainable because of the hit your pocketbook takes, is simply absurd. A basic multivitamin that houses anywhere between 30 and 60 once a day pills is anywhere between 12 and 15 US dollars on the market. Would you like to tally up how much you currently spend, take out or fast food? If you adopt the vegan lifestyle and remove animal products and dairy, then you have to make sure you replace those foods, try other fruits and experiment with other vegetables. Try to broaden your taste buds and as you do this, you will be finding other sources of vital nutrients and vitamins that were otherwise absent from your diet.

Myth number six, veganism is an eating disorder. No, no, no, no, no and no. First of all, veganism is a lifestyle, while veganism is a way of eating. Veganism is a lifestyle that seeks to exclude all forms of animal cruelty and exploitation. This includes not eating animal products and by-products, not purchasing clothing made from animal skins and boycotting news and media outlets that either support or take no stance against animal cruelty. Vegan is the eating lifestyle whereby animal products, byproducts and dairy products are removed from the diet and replaced with suitable fruits, vegetables and fortified non-dairy products in order to maintain bodily health and promote a healthy lifestyle.

An eating disorder is a mentally based condition that surfaces in physical manifestations of control, resulting in an incredibly unhealthy treatment of the body. Myth number seven, veganism is white. Apparently, some people believe that a vegan eating lifestyle and veganism in general is something that is only perpetrated and truly adopted in white upper middle class communities because of this, many people believe that vegans are somehow racist in nature, which is absolute and utter nonsense. How do I know this well? Refer back to myth number three. If you're not familiar with any of those athletes, then we will sit back and wait for you to look them up really quickly.

Did you do it well? OK, moving on, myth number eight vegans only eat eight vegetables and the food tastes horrendous. That's just insulting. Vegans eat all sorts of things, including vegetables, raw nuts, all sorts of fruits, non-dairy fortified milks and drinks, freshly squeezed juices and hemp powder proteins. They're just a few of the foods vegans take in regularly. A plant based diet is not a diet of salads. It's a diet of anything that is grown in plant form. This means potatoes, fresh herbs and spices, bananas, grapes and virtually anything else that grows on a plant is consumable on this diet. Luckily enough, these are the same ingredients that can be used to make spicy chilies, hearty stews, sweet potato lasagnas and even pizza. Now, that sounds pretty yummy to me. The

myths perpetrated in the public sector are usually myths concocted by the media. They swing stories for their benefit in an attempt to garner ratings and attention without giving any thought to the detriment they're doing to society as a whole.

Many people have been led away from adopting a vegan lifestyle because of the things they have seen on the news that are simply not true. The myths above are just a handful of the myths perpetuated over the decades since plant based diets have surged back into the public eye. And it's important to understand that these myths are not only false but preposterous. However, if debunking these myths still have you wondering if you'll be able to stay physically fit on this type of eating lifestyle, then the next chapter is for you. In this next chapter, we will outline many major athletes who have fully adopted a vegan eating lifestyle who are exponentially stronger than you.

Vegan Athletes - Plenty Of Muscle

In this chapter, we'll talk about vegan athletes with more muscles than you. Many prominent athletes have adopted vegan diets and lifestyles and have not only maintained their strength, but also promoted their inward health past a point they felt possible as a traditional eater. One of the most famous stories is, Of course, Venus Williams. In 2011, Venus was diagnosed with Shogun Syndrome, which is an autoimmune disease, and this is what prompted her to adopt a raw vegan lifestyle when her diagnosis took her out of the world of tennis. It was her adopting this type of eating lifestyle that brought her back to the court despite her autoimmune condition.

Ever since, she has trained harder, become more efficient and has stood alongside her sister, who also adapted the vegan lifestyle in order to support her sister through this uncertain road and has since stood toe to toe with her on the court. Mike Tyson is another athlete who not only stayed strong, but also kept his muscle mass even after he switched to a plant based diet when Tyson made the switch to clean living. He became an outspoken proponent of the vegan lifestyle. He dropped over 100 pounds after cutting meat and animal byproducts from his diet, and he proclaims that it has helped him with a variety of issues he began experiencing as he got older. He tells anyone who will listen that as his age started to creep up, he felt his physical condition beginning to slip.

He was experiencing arthritis, sharp joint pain and tacking on weight at an enormous rate since switching to the plant based eating and animal free lifestyle not only have those issues cleared up, but he's also gained the bulk of his energy back in the latter years of his life. Max Danzig is a prominent name in the world of Mae fighting, and he was criticized a great deal when he made the decision to adopt a plant based diet in the meat eating world of May. He now stuck out like a sore thumb while he cut the dairy out quite some time before the full movie because of allergies. He states that the primary reason he shifted to a full on plant based diet was because he felt his body was not at the peak physical condition it could have been in regards to his fighting.

Yes, a prominent M.A fighter adopted a plant based eating regimen because he wanted more from his body. Among his list of foods he eats on a regular basis, black beans, lentils and seeds topped the list. Next, we have baseball superstar Hank Aaron. Hank Aaron is just another prominent athlete in the world of athletes that adopted a plant based lifestyle in order to further their strength, agility and energy stores for their career. He is a 25 time all star in baseball and has never once argued or disputed his diet to the press. Simply the length of his illustrious and historical career tells us that not only is a plant based lifestyle good for the body, it also shows that it has no bearing on an individual's strength.

However, no list of vegan athletes is complete without the mention of Tony Gonzalez, infamous tight end in the NFL. He has openly admitted that his dietary choices have caused many awkward eyebrow raises during his career. The catalyst for his decision was a chance meeting he had on an airplane with businessman David Polaski. What happened during that encounter? Well, Polaski kept refusing standard meat and cheese dishes that were being offered to first class passengers on the plane they were both inhabiting. And Gonzalez got curious and asked why Polaski introduced him to the China study, which was an experiment performed where multiple scientists found that Chinese citizens who eat fewer animal products were less susceptible to many different illnesses.

Polaski talked with him about the theories behind many of the illnesses that plague Americans in regards to their diets. And the rest is history. Gonzalez is the billboard example for both the dangers and the benefits of adopting a vegan diet. When he first began his diet, he dropped a substantial amount of weight because he was uninformed about the nutrition side of the eating lifestyle. In essence, he cut out all animal products without replacing them with other protein, fruit and vegetable sources due to his weight loss. He lost his strength and this is when he decided to begin educating himself.

He spoke with several doctors and specialists and read every type of material he could get his hands on. And he figured out where he had gone wrong and took every effort to change it. He quickly began incorporating more plant protein sources he didn't know existed, and it put him back in fighting shape within a few short months. So what is this plant based diet done for his career? Well, since adopting the diet, he has not only become incredibly outspoken about his decisions because of the criticism many in the NFL gave him, which have led many individuals to adopt vegan eating habits of their own. He's also set several athletic records within his career, including a career reception record for his position in football.

The truth of the matter is that adopting a plant based lifestyle, if done right and with the right amount of knowledge, can help your body heal. Not only that, but it can also help to strengthen your body in ways that traditional eating lifestyle cannot, because the variety of foods you have to adopt will also come jam packed with macro and micronutrients. Your body is not getting otherwise. So with all of this in mind, what does a vegan eat? Do they take supplements anyway? What type of foods have those sources of protein and calcium that are so vital to bone and muscle health? Trust me, there is more variety than you realize.

Fueling The Vegan Warrior

In this chapter, we'll learn about fueling the vegan warrior, a vegan eating lifestyle includes the ingestion of fruits, vegetables, grains, dried beans, peas, lentils, seeds and nuts. Vegans do not consume dairy, eggs, meat, poultry, fish or any products that contain any of these foods. Many people struggle with adopting a vegan lifestyle because they believe deficiencies in calcium, iron, zinc and a host of other vital vitamins and nutrients will take place. And in part, they are right if they do not replace what they've removed with other sources of these vitamins and minerals.

If a traditional eater removes all dairy and animal products from their diet and simply eats regularly despite that removal, they are not only going to be deficient in vitamins and minerals, they will be deficient in protein and caloric intake. There are plenty of vegan sources of these very important macro and micronutrients you can plug into your diet once removing dairy and animal byproducts in order to plug in the holes those food items will cause. Protein is a vital component to building muscle, keeping strong and making sure red blood cells are healthy. It's also the component that supports growth all through a species life cycle. Sources for protein for vegans include soy and soy based products such as Tempa, fortified soy beverages and tofu veggie burgers, legumes, which is black beans, kidney beans, black eyed peas and lentils.

Grains like quinoa, oatmeal and brown rice and seeds like sunflower and sesame and nut butters irons are another vital component of a healthy diet because it helps carry oxygen to different parts of the body. It is said that vegans usually need twice the amount of iron in their diet as traditional eaters because the iron sources from plants are not as well absorbed as the iron from animal foods. But that does not mean a vegan eating lifestyle is a bad thing. The foods that contain iron also contain high amounts of micronutrients that most all other people are consistently deficient in. Sources for iron include soy and soy based products, veggie burgers, prune juice, dried apricots, cooked spinach, cooked kale, potatoes with the skin on pinto beans, azuki beans, lentils, fortified grain products, cashews, almonds and blackstrap molasses.

One thing to keep in mind with absorbing iron while eating vegan is the fact that it absorbs better when it is ingested. When paired with foods that are rich in vitamin C, these types of foods include grapefruits, oranges, kiwis, lemons, limes, potatoes, sweet peppers, broccoli and cantaloupe. And yes, their juices also count. If you are a juicer, vitamin B 12 is yet another vitamin that many would be deficient in if they did not replace those foods removed from their diet. This vitamin helps the body to utilize stored fats as well as create red blood cells.

Good sources of vitamin B 12 for a vegan include Red Star, nutritional yeast, fortified soy beverages and fortified meat alternatives like meatless, chicken and veggie burgers. Vitamin D is necessary for the body because it not only helps to stave off seasonal depression and help regulate the brain's chemistry, but it also AIDS in the absorption and conversion of phosphorus and calcium into usable components that aid in strong teeth and bones. Vegan sources of vitamin D include non hydrogenated margarines and fortified vegan friendly products. Also the sun cat outside and get yourself some sun.

Speaking of calcium, this is another one of the controversial nutrients that vegans supposedly do not get enough of. Calcium is necessary for bone and muscle health and helps with muscular contractions like your heartbeat. There are numerous calcium sources for vegans, and some of them are soy yogurt, fortified, non-dairy beverages, navy beans, sesame butter, also called tahini, blackstrap molasses, bok choy, okra, figs and fortified orange juice. Zinc is another mineral many people are deficient in, and there are many sources of it. For those who choose a vegan eating lifestyle, zinc is necessary for basic development and growth, and it also AIDS in strengthening the immune system and healing wounds inflicted upon the body.

Good sources of zinc for vegans include peas, lentils, and dried beans. Pecans, cashew butter, peanut butter, pumpkin seeds and fortified whole grains. The last nutrient that many people are deficient in that can be provided on a vegan diet is linolenic acid. If you don't recognize that name, then you will probably recognize it by its other name. Omega three fatty acids. Omega 3s are important for nerve, eye and brain development, but are also helpful in preventing heart disease and cardiac events. There are some wonderful vegan friendly sources, some of which include flaxseed oil, soybean oil, canola oil, ground, flaxseed tofu and walnuts.

But if you're an athlete or workout intensively while adopting a vegan eating lifestyle, then supplements are usually something worked into the health regimen no matter what. Vegans, however, have to be very careful with the types of supplements they choose to take. Many supplements on the market have animal byproduct additives to aid in its preservation and shelf life, and it can wreak havoc on a vegan's body if they have gone for an extended period of time without consuming animal products or byproducts. If you find yourself to be a picky eater, then all of the nutrients and vitamins previously listed would be wonderful. To work into your morning or evening routine, just make sure you find a vegan friendly distributor of these vitamins to stay within the boundaries of your diet.

For most vegans, a basic vegan certified multivitamin that includes B 12 will be enough. Those multivitamins show zinc, iodine, vitamin C, omega three fatty acids, as well as a slew of micronutrients that your body can benefit from. However, if you are someone who is eating a vegan lifestyle and training or working out regularly, then it's recommended you find a branched chain amino acid that is vegan friendly in order to help your body recuperate from the beating your muscles are taking in your workout chapters. These B.C. A's will help your body to maintain the muscles it's breaking down and strengthening instead of you simply losing your strength.

It will also aid in keeping your bones strong during training as well. The truth of the matter is that dropping entire food groups from your body, while healthier, will inevitably create holes in the nutrients you're receiving. Our stereotypical dietary pyramid that kids are taught in school is not focused on keeping their body entirely healthy for the long run. But it's there to make sure they get the right amount of vitamins and minerals daily. In other words, our dietary pyramid is not constructed with bodily health in mind, but with nutrient health in mind. And yes, there is a difference. This means that supplements will be necessary. How will you know if you need supplements? Start by finding a basic vegan friendly multivitamin.

You can take daily and a vegan friendly BKE if you're working out and training regularly and see how your body feels from there. If there is a list outlined above whose foods you simply cannot stomach, then that is an individual nutrient and or vitamin that will probably require its own bulk daily supplement. But now that you have all this information, it's time to tackle the last informational part of this chapter. Of course, before we talk about going vegan and what that entails, this last part is addressing the intimidating work of exercise and what it means and looks like to someone who eats a vegan diet.

Vegan Warrior Workout Plan

In this chapter, we'll learn about the Vegan Warrior workout plan, getting him becoming active can be difficult for many people, no matter the diet they take on a lack of motivation, morbid obesity, time restraints and other issues make it very easy for people to either not have the time or not find the energy to become motivated to move. Each person has a unique case and there's no single solution that fits everyone. However, if you have chosen to adopt the vegan diet, then you have already taken one step in the right direction for the health of your body for the long term. This means the next major step is going to be figuring out what sort of workout plan you want to utilize.

A very common way for beginners to start exercising is to take an easy start. This usually means going outside and walking for short 10 minute bursts or taking the plunge to get that gym membership and going and walking on a treadmill for 15 minutes. For people who want to do some sort of muscle training, you can do particular exercises within the comfort of your own home. Another important facet is to keep motivated during your exercising. The most popular way to keep motivated is via music. But you can also utilize television in order to help you develop the habit of regular exercise.

The whole point of beginning an exercise journey on a vegan diet is making sure to ingrain the habit in order to complete your path in the journey towards better health. You have to choose some sort of workout plan. This will be a plan that you follow week by week that can be easily tailored upwards as your body becomes more efficient in utilizing its energy and becomes generally stronger. Even though you're eating a vegan lifestyle, all of your muscle groups in some way need to be exercised. This includes your abdomen, your thighs and all the muscles in your back and arms. Simply doing nothing but cardio is not going to make you stronger, and it's not an efficient use of the calories you are giving your body. One of the things people have to keep in mind when exercising on a vegan diet is that you're going to have to feed your body more in order to keep up your energy.

Traditional eaters consume massive amounts of protein indicative to the size of their workout program because protein from animal sources stays in the body longer. This means that an individual who eats meat and animal byproducts could go to a restaurant and have a nice meal, then still have that fuel two hours later when they decide to go to the gym. Vegans do not have that kind of convenience because plant based sources of protein are not as easily absorbed into the body, nor are they held onto for as long as meat based sources of protein. This means that some sort of energy has to be given to the body within 30 minutes of the exercise you choose to do.

Not only that, but you usually have to replenish that store of energy after you workout. This does not mean you have to eat an entire meal before and after your workout. This simply means that a snack, a juice or a shake of some sort should be ingested 30 minutes before and no later than 30 minutes after your workout. Cardio is an imperative part of a workout regimen for a vegan because it will help to keep your blood sugar levels at bay with the amount of carbohydrate you take in on this type of diet. The thing about a vegan diet is that even though it eliminates food groups, it does not designate a specific amount of caloric or carbohydrate intake that has to be eaten throughout the day.

So cardio and all of its offshoots are going to help an individual regulate their blood sugars when trying to figure out the appropriate caloric intake for their body. Things like 15 minute walks outside, 15 minute walks on the treadmill, 30 minutes of swimming, cycling classes and even yoga tapes you can do in the comfort of your own home all count as legitimate sources of cardio. You should be implementing at least three times a week strength training for your muscles and your bones also need to be incorporated into your workout. And it should be anywhere between 30 and 45 minutes each time you go to do it.

The reason you don't want to go over forty five minutes is because it can be over-exhausting to the muscle groups you're working and it can cause damage that will keep you from exercising. You do not want to hit all of the muscle groups more than twice a week because this will also ensure that you keep an even muscle development over all the muscles of your body without overworking and hurting yourself. For those of you who are just beginning their strength training, you can do simple weightlifting in the comfort of your own home. You can also do body weight, squats and catchphrases to work the lower half of your body.

Things like push ups and sit ups will work. Your arms and your upper back, as well as your abdomen and planks are really good. Way to engage every single muscle of your body, and they can all be done in the comfort of your own home, strength training is a little more fluid in how often to implement it throughout the week because it's less tailored to the number of times you simply do it and more tailored to the number of times you've worked out a specific group of your body. Remember, during the week for strength training, you have to make sure you work every muscle of your body twice, whether you are situated. So you are strength training every day or whether you are situated.

So your strength training three times a week, it doesn't matter. What matters is the length of time you strength train and the duration you touch on those major muscle groups every week. There are other ways you can incorporate working out into your lifestyle that are less traditional and more convenient to familiar lifestyles. Sports, climbing a tree with your kids or your family. Gymnastics and resistance bands are all wonderful ways to enhance your workout plan without stepping into a gym. There are also certain classes you could take out in the community that have the potential to get you around many other like minded individuals, such as martial arts and kickboxing. These avenues are great because they do not only incorporate cardio and strength training, but they also enhance the strength of your bones.

Now it's time for the most important part of the Book. Up until this point, you have merely been fed information. You've been instructed on the guidelines that eating a vegan diet affords. You have been instructed on the types of exercising you can implement. And you've even witnessed thus debunk multiple myths that come with the vegan diet that have been misinterpreted and perpetuated by society. It is now time to go over how to correctly and safely implement this change in your life so you have the greatest chance of succeeding.

Going Vegan

In this chapter, we'll talk about going vegan, the first step for any new lifestyle change is to do your research. However, we've already done the heavy lifting for you, so you've decided to take the plunge into a vegan way of eating. You've cleared out your home of all animal products and byproducts and filled your home with lots of things, according to the food list outlined previously. So now what? Understanding one thing. Your body is not supposed to be hungry. If you are giving your body ample amounts of healthy food filled with nutrients, you will lose weight easily, 4000 calories of fast food and 4000 calories of fresh fruits, vegetables and legumes are two completely different things.

And your body will lose weight by instilling the latter rather than the former. Don't think that adopting a vegan diet in order to lose weight or help your long term health means going hungry. Grab a snack if you get hungry in between meals. Awareness is also a vital part of going vegan. Listening to your body and interpreting what it wants is imperative to being able to give it the nutrients it's longing for on a daily basis. For most people, it's easy to distinguish between when the body is thirsty and when it's hungry. However, for many of those other people, it could be hard when the body becomes hungry, but has no particular craving for it. Becoming in tune with your body and being able to interpret its needs via the brain signals that are being shot throughout your system is vital to becoming a vegan.

Not only that, it's vital to becoming a well-adjusted individual. For many, implementing a lifestyle is not something you can just do. As in, jumping in feet first will always lead them down a path of failure. If you are the type of person who could throw out or donate all the food in your kitchen, refill it and start your new eating lifestyle full force tomorrow, then you are more likely to succeed. But not everyone is like that. For those who are not like that, here's something you can do. Go through your kitchen and take stock of everything that is not going to be kosher for a vegan eating lifestyle. All meats, refined sugars, snacks and animal byproducts need to be written down on the list.

Then you need to put this list somewhere where you'll be able to see it every day. Now, every time you go grocery shopping, cross two items off that list that you will not purchase and refill your kitchen with and instead replace it with something for your new plant based diet that you will incorporate regularly into your kitchen. For example, if you're ditching the chips and salsa, then opt for something crunchy like carrots and then purchase all the ingredients needed to make your own salsa. Another tip is to eat before you go shopping. If you go into a grocery store hungry, it is going to be much harder sticking to your vegan shopping list.

If you are constantly passing by the junk food and candy aisles, it's also going to behoove you, at least for the first few trips, to write out your grocery list and take it with you. Whether you jot it down in your phone or whether you write it out physically on a piece of paper, having that accountability right in front of you is going to help you stay on track. Making these small changes in your diet is going to help you instill the diet for the long haul, resulting in long term health advances that will not only help you lose weight, but will help advance the efficiency of your body as well as heal your organs and immune system. It takes time to adapt to a diet change such as this one. So make sure you take it in stride.

Understand that 70 percent of this process is mental and it's overcoming those mental barriers that will help you to get to a point where a vegan eating lifestyle is not simply a diet, but a new way of life. Some daily habits you can begin implementing are making up snacks prior to wanting them meal, planning your week, designating one day a week to go grocery shopping and to always keep trying new foods and learning. Making your snacks prior to wanting them will help keep you from jeopardizing your new way of eating by grabbing something more convenient and meal planning, your week will help you keep from falling prey to the convenience of takeout. Not only that, but designating one day a week to grocery shop will help your wallet because you'll be able to use all the fresh products you purchased before.

It wilts and goes bad. A vegan diet in the long run is actually easier on your wallet if you can minimize food waste by shopping every week instead of every paycheck. But the most important thing is to always keep learning. Purchase a book every so often on the vegan diet and read through it to see if there's any new information. Do research on exotic fruits and vegetables. You can try at that new restaurant that just opened up downtown and listen to other vegan athletes and prominent vegan individuals to see what works for them, just like any other way of eating veganism.

And the vegan diet is not a static entity. Eating the same things day in and day out without ever trying new things or implementing new tactics is going to get boring. Not only that, it can create massive nutritional holes in your diet. Stick to these steps and habits necessary for implementing a vegan diet and you're well on your way to improving your long term health, losing weight, aiding the environment, and even tapping into a store of strength and energy you did not realize you could have.

Thoughts & Tips

Thank you again for reading this chapter . Becoming a vegan warrior is all about strength, mental acuity and determination. It takes dedication as well as knowledge to properly and healthfully act a vegan lifestyle. So make sure you never stop learning about the diet and all it entails. There are many myths floating out there that misappropriate and perpetuate false information when it comes to a vegan lifestyle. If you are nervous about having to take supplements, then understand this. Traditional eaters are the biggest consumers of supplements on the market.

Why? Because despite them eating animal products and by-products, they are still deficient in their intake of vitamins and minerals because of a massive reduction in fruits and vegetables. Many traditional eaters are under the assumption that animal products and byproducts will give them everything they need, and that is simply not true. Not only do traditional eaters usually take in too much protein, they are drained of their energy stores because of a lack of proper nutrition. Yes, becoming a vegan in diet and in lifestyle helps the environment, but that is not the only reason to adopt this diet.

Several research studies that have been conducted have paired a vegan diet up against many other diets, such as vegetarian, a traditional diet, a low carbohydrate diet, a high fat diet, and even a high protein diet. Not only did participants in a vegan diet lose nine point three more pounds on average than any other person on any other diet tested, they also saw a drastic balancing of their blood sugar levels, their heart rate and their blood pressure. Do not allow anyone to convince you that going vegan is going to somehow ruin your strength.

The Williams sisters, professional NFL football players, boxers and even male athletes are just a few among the thousands of athletes who eat a plant based diet. Many of those athletes have discovered strength they did not know they had and have told people time and time again that they would never have unlocked that strength and fortitude if they had not adapted to a plant based eating lifestyle. Protein is not the end all be all of strength. It takes massive amounts of micro and macro nutrients in order to upkeep your muscles and bones at a cellular level. A diverse vegan diet gives you plenty of those so you can stay healthy in the gym.

And all of those micro and macro nutrients also offer you more energy. So recuperation from the gym and from any other workout regimen is going to be a bit quicker. Exercising is something you need to implement on a vegan diet, whether you take a walk for 15 minutes every day or you begin your journey down a two hour workout regimen in order to build and toned muscle, you need to make sure two things occur. You need to make sure it is a steady plan you can handle and you need to make sure all of the facets of your health are being exercised. What this means is just cardio or just weight lifting is not going to work. There has to be a healthy combination of both in order to really succeed exercising while adopting a vegan eating lifestyle.

The most popular way to do this is to workout six times a week with three days being cardio based and three days being muscle based. That cardio can range anywhere from a walk around your block to swimming for an hour. And that strength training can range anywhere from doing sit ups and push ups in your own home to going into the gym and utilizing their weight machines. Whatever you choose to do and whatever you find works for you, stick to it. I hope this chapter, Of course, simply educated you and helped you feel more comfortable with the idea of eating vegan. The next step is to implement whether you take one step at a time or you start full throttle tomorrow. The next step is physical implementation. And I promise you, you can do this. You are stronger than you realize.

Body & Mind Health Masterclass: A Complete Guide to BodyDetox

Let me ask you a question. How would you like to go back to the days of a teenager. How would you like to feel young and vibrant? How would you like your body to be flexible and react to every move that you take without any resistance? Welcome to our body detox Book. In this Book you are going to witness nothing less than a miracle. Millions of people around the planet are eating, sleeping and going about their daily lives unconsciously with no idea what they're actually doing to their bodies. We are not taught how to eat, how to sleep, how to be parents and how to manage our finances. These are not things that we learned in school. These are things that we are required to learn as we go. And this Book by taking this Book. It's one of the best decisions you will ever take in your lifetime. Guaranteed. Take it from someone who's been through this destock detox process many many times and each time I go through this process I'm amazed at the effect that has on my life.

People around me are just amazed at the change in just a few days. People come up to you and they say you know something about you. Your skin is different. Have you put makeup on? It's neat. These kinds of questions you know that they're not ready yet. They happen and you say to them Well I just did a detox Book because you're sleeping better because your memory is better you have more vitality you have more energy at all the toxins are leaving your body your stomach shrinks all the body fat just slowly leaves your body and you are left with just the body of your dreams. This is something that is a reality. It's possible. And it's very simple if you just follow the Book as we take you along you'll see that by the end of this Book you'll be a different person guaranteed. So let's begin.

Expectations & Days 1-3

To reach this result this destination this prize that we're aiming for there is a road that we need to go down and it's not going to be easy for the first few days but once we pass this obstacle of the first few days you will see that it will just be second nature to you because the first few days what is happening is your body can go into shock and you know what's going on. It's used to all these calves and sugars and caffeine to get through the day and you're basically denying your body of what it is craving or what it thinks that it needs in order to thrive. So what's going to happen is for the first few days it may be a little challenging but once we get past these few days you'll see how quickly your body is gonna react to change and it's going to be incredible and every second every minute that passes you will see a change in your body how it reacts and how it no longer craves the sugars and the carbs and it's just a journey that is worth taking because after one two three or four days time you will the compliments start flowing and you start.

People say you're looking incredible. There's something different about you. You'll be waking up in the morning with more energy. You'll be smiling more, you'll be a happier person, you'll be more pleasant to be around, maybe less rage, maybe less shouting at the kids, the wife or random people at the supermarket. Think of it this way during the first three days you will be dropped not literally in the middle of a desert and all you are giving is rice and unlimited amounts of water. What we are limiting in our diet is sugar and salt, spices and caffeine. So basically these are cut out of our diet and what we are doing now is we are taking the rice and the qualities of the fiber of the rice are basically killing that they are cleaning the pack out of our intestines and also the and also the dull taste of the rice is resetting our taste buds which is so used to that beautiful taste of sugar and chocolate and sweets and all those yummy things that have to be cut out now for the next few days unfortunately.

But there is a great prize at the end so let's carry on to the next stage. One more thing that I forgot to say is about the stickiness of the rice. Now some people like their rice. Exactly done according to the recipe at the stickiness amount that we are choosing in this Book is more towards the stickiness of sushi which basically teaches us to chew properly chew our food properly slowly as we are meant to chew not just from our rubber or Rod Paige or go through all our food as quickly as possible. This is a conscious process and it's something that requires a little bit of practice but after a few days it'll be second nature. Also another thing that we are going to get used to is to drink half an hour before or half an hour after our meal not with our meal just like you don't put water in your gas tank. You refrain from drinking while you are eating so that the food is allowed to digest properly and once it's digested then we can take those fluids and the body will react and that is what we are digesting.

Enemas

One of the most recommended turbo charges to this process that I personally recommend not for everyone is an enema. Now the big E word a lot of people know at this point will kind of freak out but let me say this. I was also very anti animals or any kind of penetrating procedures. But the first time I did it it was a complete life changer for me. Life changer. This process is harmless. In fact it's so beneficial that it will just take you to another level. Let me just explain the meaning behind the animal. During our lifetime when all these toxins are basically accumulating in our system they serve as a base for all the parasites to breed in our system. They cause bellies to enlarge and they cause a lot of health issues and they refrain all the good nutrients and vitamins from entering our system. And they basically just wreak havoc.

A lot of toxins accumulate in our intestines and they cause most of our health issues. And this is what also causes you to know all the desire for sweets and for carbs and all those cravings that we have. This is due to all the accumulation of all the toxins that are basically in our body and we need to clean that stuff out. Even though you are brushing your teeth every single day, maybe twice a day, you still need to go and see that dentist because of all those little parts in your mouth that you can't get them out by yourself even if you're flossing. You still need to go to the dentist. This is exactly the same. And even more important because you can't see it. And because this affects your entire system. OK. So what I want to emphasize here is the importance of this enema. If you want to turbo charge this process I highly recommend it. If not we will continue anyway. And there are other alternatives which I will present to you.

Days 4-8

On day number four we will introduce the carrot and this will be at the light for our taste buds because we haven't been accustomed to anything sweet and the natural sweetness of the carrots will be delicious for us. The carrot is great because what it does is it resets the functioning of the spleen which when it's not functioning properly will cause all kinds of mucus and also a bed for parasites and all kinds of issues in our health system. So the current helps to reset the system. It's a great visual to bring into our detox the day afterwards. They number five we will introduce the pumpkin and the pumpkin as well. We'll just feel like it's the first time that you've tasted this special. It will be like you're eating candy because the natural taste of a pumpkin is so delicious and sweet that you haven't even tried it in your lifetime. Only when you were a baby.

So it's been a very long time since you've tasted these vegetables with your palate reset in such a way that you will enjoy the vegetable as it was meant to be enjoyed on day number six and seven will we will be introducing celery and parsley and these two vegetables full of salt these sorts of vital for our body to function well and they will give us an indication of how much salt we were consuming beforehand and whether you know this or not salts in moderation is OK. But too much salt increases our blood pressure and it causes us to inflate. So after a week of vegetables which we've been eating by the way we will be sorting them or we can eat them raw whichever is your preference. I personally like to diversify my pie detox diet.

Sometimes I have to grow up, sometimes I like to steam them everyone. Each to their own.

After seven days of these vegetables we will introduce the protein. This is where the party starts because we've been a week without protein people. We got to feel a little bit tired and exhausted, maybe depending on how you're reacting. And as you know our bodies require protein in order to get the fuel that it needs in order to get through the day in order to process all that energy. So day by day we'll be introducing another type of protein until we find which one is right for us which one isn't right for us. And this is just this is just a process of trial and error basically because your body is now cleaner than before. Every food that reacts to your body in a manner that is not in complete harmony with your system will tell us immediately whether it's right for you or whether it is.

Energy levels

For those of you who are concerned about your levels of energy do not worry because during this period we are going to supplement our diet with chlorophyll and with super green plants these the combination of these two will basically help us fill the give us the energy that we are required to require for us to go about our daily lives. Just like a bull in nature who eats feeds of greens he doesn't get huge into that amount of muscle from feeding on meat. So what we're doing is we're going to take the chlorophyll out of the super green blends. Don't worry I will direct you to the best resources and the best place to find online. And these two supplements will help us cleanse our body, increase our levels of iron and of Uncle Ben and will also help us to clear out all the toxins from our body and continue with the process. Best way possible.

Restarting the System

Every day we are going to add to our plan a new spice and a new hope. And we're going to discover on our bodies just like a chart just like a baby who is coming off the breastfeeding that the mother does straight away. Feed him hamburgers and coke. Slowly we introduce new foods to the baby and we see how the baby reacts to various foods and you know something's bothering the baby and there's an allergic reaction. Then we eliminate that food and we go through the whole scale of foods until we reach the right amount to the right variety of foods which is good for our baby. So in the same way what we're doing here in our time is introducing new spices, new herbs, and new foods. Slowly, we will discover what works for us and what doesn't.

Because this is something that we've taken for granted just like if you fill up your gas instead of in your car you put diesel inside of your car straight away the engine is gonna go crazy and you need to take it to the mechanic. This is the same way in our bodies we've lost connection to our bodies all these years we don't know what's working for us, what's causing us what. So by resetting our system introducing new foods we can then reconnect and discover the right foods for us by agreeing with what's disagreeing with us.

And just like a baby we will basically be at peace again with our bodies in harmony and our diet will be the right for us now from this stage onwards we will be consuming various supplements dietary supplements according to precise instructions from me you will take these supplements in order to supercharge this detox and get rid of all the parasites and the toxins out of the body and make this detox the most efficient that we can because that is our purpose. As soon as we get rid of all these parasites out of our body which we've been unaware of until today you will notice that all the cravings for the sugar and perhaps even the body excess body weight will just disappear like it's never been and you will notice a huge change in your day to day activities.

Parasite Home Test

What I'm going to tell you now is the best way to find out if you have parasites in your body. First thing in the morning when you wake up and take a glass of water and you spit into the glass of water providing you haven't cleaned your teeth or used any mouthwash. And after five minutes you notice in the cup if the saliva has disappeared or if a kind of jellyfish has formed in the glass. If the jellyfish is formed inside the glass then congratulations you have parasites in your body. If the saliva has disappeared from your home free and what we want to do is within a month or a month and a half we want to reach the ideal goal of having a pink tub with clean no black or white flag on the top and no cut down the middle. It's gonna be a beautiful pink top and that our species will be clean and it will be how it's supposed to be. Please excuse me for the terminology but it's supposed to be one piece. No smell, no dirt on the toilet paper. That's my friends. It's the sign of a clean body.

Elimination

Listen, the word diet has picked up a bad name in past years. It has a connotation of punishment. And you know what it really means is finding the right nutrition, the right foods that are good for you that are working for you as an individual. And nothing here is extreme. No diet should be extreme. What we're doing here is a process of elimination and we're finding the right foods that are good for us even though during the first couple of weeks we will be following a strict plan. The whole essential idea behind this detox plan is to regain confidence in your body and to find out what is working for you, what causes you to thrive and what foods are causing you discomfort. And this is vital. This is the essential part of our plan. OK. Like I said this process is not easy but it is worth it.

I guarantee you at the end of this process you will be a different person. If you have any questions feel free to send us any questions that you may have Facebook or through the phone and we will do our best to answer you as quickly as possible so even though I haven't met you in person I'm proud of you for taking this journey. It's a bold one that not many people choose to take but I guarantee you that on the other side there is a whole new world waiting for you to discover.

An Emotional & Physical Journey

You know I've witnessed hundreds of people who've been through this process including myself. I can tell you from my experience that when we go through a physical cleansing it's also an emotional cleansing. If we have toxins in our liver then we also have emotional toxins in our liver And what parasites are are basically they are an external force which is managing our lives. And instead of us managing our body our body is managing us. So what I've come to see throughout the years is that when we cleanse and all the toxins leave our body we begin to release emotions you know anger fear anxiety people that we didn't want in our lives. They suddenly leave because it's part of the process.

And what happens is that we begin to restart our system and we begin to let go of things that we've been holding onto for so many years. And you can really feel this happening especially especially when you're doing the enema you will experience visualizations of things that happened to you when you were five when you were 7-10. All kinds of situations and you will release them back into the universe and you will be free again because these things have been managing you they're sitting inside your body and you'll live in your subconscious mind and they've been running your life. It's time to let it go. And this is basically what I'm saying is it's a physical journey and an emotional journey too.

Products required

The materials we need for our detox process are as follows: two kilos of home short grain rice. We've already discussed the properties of whole grain rice and how it cleans our insides. Very very very well. We need three to four kilos of lemons. The lemons will serve us in our animal process. Those of you who decide to do the animal process lemon cleans limescale. As you know from kennels from kitchen appliances. So it also cleanses our body and the plaque inside and what it does. It just washes out all the toxins out during the enema so it's a very vital product when we use the enema. Another product that we need in our enema is camomile. We'll need about 50 grams of camomile flowers. We can use a camomile tea bag which is just a camomile with no green tea, no caffeine, no additives , just pure Melba.

Obviously the preference is for flowers while the camomile does. This infects it suits and comes and it works in harmony with the lemon during the enema. Another product that we need is coffee. Now some places in the world coffee changes the type of coffee that you can buy. The best type of coffee that we recommend for the enema is black coffee Turkish coffee. If you couldn't find it because the texture of the Turkish coffee is very, you know the texture of it is the right density for the cleansing of the liver and the cleansing for the toxins that will be released during the enema. So if you can find Turkish coffee great if you'd prefer just regular black coffee that's great as well. We will need a home enema kit which you can buy online.

It should be a two liter capacity. You can buy it online on various websites. Obviously we'll share with you the links at the end of the chapter. On the page of course you will find links to various websites that sell very easily and it's very important that the kit that you buy leads to a kit. This is the capacity that we are looking for. Another product that we need in our cleansing is super green. Mix this blend also which we will provide links to where to find them online. This blend provides us with a great supplement in the detox process with a cleansing of the toxins out and providing all vs the vitamins and minerals and the essential nutrients that we need when we are cleaning our body and providing us with the energy that we require. You know when we're doing all this detox process the next material that we need is the or we're going to oil the oregano oil is considered by some the holy grail of antibiotic natural natural antibiotics for many many different for a whole wide range of complaints and situations.

The original oil should be bought as Mediterranean oregano oil and it should have at least 70 percent concentration now over going to oil. We will also explain how it can be taken. For some it's very spicy and bitter but there are various ways to take the regional oil and water underneath the tongue and it does its job so it's worth it. We also need an enzyme digestive mix. This will help us with digestion and the absorption of the minerals and vitamins in our system which we have damaged due to our lifestyle. We also need a powerful probiotic mix between 25 to 50 billion bacteria strains of bacteria is what we're looking for and this is something that will help balance our good and bad bacteria in our system and help boost our immune system. So probiotics are a very important product in our detox cleansing process. And in general we should always be taking probiotics to balance our system.

Defecation

One of the main changes that we will see during the process is in the defecation that our stool and poop is going to change. Now this is because of the fact that we are changing our diet. OK it's not constipation we will be going less to the toilet. This is not constipation. So no need to worry. But there may be some aches or some nauseousness that accompany this process and this is natural because basically our body is breaking down the fact that it needs energy. So if you need to take something chemical, if it's a pill, something to feel better go ahead. You know it's not something that we recommend because this is a natural process and we want to keep it as natural as possible. But if you feel that is something that is bothering you and it's impacting your process then go ahead and you know we want to feel better. OK. So if you feel that you do need to take something.

Go ahead. But I just wanted to let you know that this is natural. OK. There are a lot of toxins that are being surfaced and they are being washed out of our system. This is why we are feeling the way we do. It's natural they are leaving our gut though leaving our system through the lymphatic system through the other various organs. So it's natural to feel various side effects. So just be at ease with it and let the process happen within four or five days. The symptoms will disappear and the process will take on a kind of rhythm and you'll start to feel a lot better. Energy levels will rise, you'll start to sleep better, have more energy, and you'll breathe better your taste buds. Believe me you'll be able to smell your neighbor's food better than you've ever surmounted before your girlfriend, boyfriend , wife , friends , and roommates will stop complaining about your snoring. So let's move on.

Changes

Also you will notice on the emotional side of things how the changes will begin to affect your life. There'll be a little bit more lightness, a bit more happiness, more joy, maybe a more positive outlook on life. People start to compliment you perhaps on how your skin is radiating just the other day. During my detox process someone said to me looks like you've just come back from vacation. I haven't been on vacation. I've just done an enema. OK. Your mood swings may change a little bit. You may start to feel a little bit lighter, a bit more excited about things, a bit more clarity, maybe your memory is improving. Usually after animals sometimes they may be a drop or there may be a rise depending on what kind of person you are. But just to let you know that these changes are normal and they're actually desirable because what we're looking to do is to reset our system.

Preparation

The evening before the detox process begins, what we suggest is that you do an enema to clean out the system and empty the waste toxins from your body. Those of you who decide to do the enema and I strongly suggest that you do then the evening before we boil two liters of water and have them at room temperature and then we will do the enema and proceed with the detox process. Now that we have a link here down below and a PDA file that you can download with all the instructions on how to do the enema properly. Step by step. But if you have any fears. If this is something that doesn't relate to you right now then that's okay too. And you can proceed without them.

Documenting process

It's very very important that we now document where we are before we start the process. One of the best tips that I can give you is that if you document how you are looking now and how you will look when you finish you will be able to see the huge difference. And it actually starts after a day or two. I am currently after a week of my annual detox process and I can tell you I've already lost a few kilos and it's something that you can see clearly when you film it in a very well documented in a very precise manner. What I mean is basically you just take a photo of yourself or have someone take a photo of yourself a full body photo and you should also take a photo of your time. You should basically take your tongue out like this.

Take a photo of your tongue. This is because we want to document the change in our tongue. At the beginning it will be a little bit discolored. There's some change in the shape of our time and as we do our detox process that the shape of the indent in our town and the discovery will change which is why it's important to document it at the beginning so we can tell the difference and we can see as we go along the great progress that we are making.

First days

We begin the morning with a spoonful of chlorophyll in a glass of water. This will provide us with some energy for those of you who could not get through the morning without the coffee. It will also help with a detox process and with the iron account in our system the super Herb blend mix will provide us also with a boost of the detox process and will reduce our feelings of hunger and we'll also clean out the toxins and provide us with the vitamins that we need. Just like Popeye the Sailor Man and his famous spinach. Over the next three days we will be eating rice and rice and more rice. Basically the menu is compiled from rice.

What we want to do is boil the rice with three cups of water, bring it to a boil and then we throw one cup of rice into the water and bring it to a boil. Lower the heat and then let it simmer for 30 to 40 minutes until all the water has absorbed and the rice comes out a little bit mushy which is the ratio of three to one when usually we're doing two to one. So the reason for this is that we want the rice to be more edible. We want it to be basically we want to chew slower. We want to. We want to get used to chewing slowly slowly so that we will fill up our stomachs at a better rate and we will be basically consuming less carbs in this method.

Our taste buds are now being reset as we are used to our food being consumed with sugar and salt. The two main ingredients that cause us to gain weight it is actually the outer shell of the rice which is serving as a basically a dentist an inner toothbrush which is scratching off the plaque from the insides of our system which is refrain which is basically preventing the absorption of the good minerals and vitamins into our system. And that is what is making us feel tired and lethargic with low levels of energy and then obviously we go to the sugar and the carbs and the coffee to raise our levels of energy again and the cycle goes on and on and on. So after the first day of our delicious meals of rice we will do an enema in the evening of water for those of you who decide to do the enema on the second day of the delicious meals of rice.

We will also do an enema in the evening to clean out the toxins. Remember this all these rice meals are without any herbs and spices and sugar and salt just the rice. There is no limit no limits to how much rice you can consume the amount of meals that you have. So feel free to eat rice all day long. On the third day we will do the fourth NMR which will be with a camomile and the lemon to basically disinfect and soothe our system after we've been eating to survive and detoxifying our system. Now one very important note regarding the eating process. I strongly advise that if you drink water when you're thirsty it is half an hour before you eat the rice and an hour after you eat the rice. Because this is how we do not interfere with the enzymes which are responsible for the absorption of all the good minerals in our stomach and will leave us feeling tired and fabric full bloated etc..

Preparation for enema

This is regarding the NRMA. And although this can be a scary process for many people what I say is that what's scaring is actually that the thought of it because although we are kind of interfering with the natural process of the body what we want to do is we want to return to the natural state that we were before we ruined it with all the sugars and carbs and all the junk that we filled ourselves up with the process of the anima although it is external. It's really not a big deal because you know the size of what we're actually inserting is smaller than what comes out of our bodies every single day. So if we're looking at that fact alone then the physical side of it is really not that bad. It's what we think about it and how we address the animal in our minds.

That is what is scary to some people which is why if you think about it thousands of people have actually gone through this process and they've come out the other side feeling much much better which is why if you realize that this is how it is that thousands of people have gone through this process with us for and they've come out the other side feeling great you are no different from them and which there's no reason why you shouldn't succeed as well in this process. Now when we're doing the enema it's a good idea to focus on something appealing, something happy and go to your happy place.

If it's the beach if it's some place you've been before the outdoors you know some maybe some occasion that happened during your life that helps you to relax and then once the fluids are flowing into our body it will take just a number of minutes before we fill up with the fluids and then we can go and wash out all the toxins. Now what happens sometimes is that during the first enema we feel sometimes a bit of pressure, sometimes a bit of nausea because all the toxins are coming out at once. So what a good idea for me. Sometimes people will just go to the toilet and will feel the need to go to the toilet and to let it all wash out before the animal is over which is OK because it's your first time you know. So ease off with the pressure. The second time will be easier. It will go much smoother. The third time you will become a lot better at this process.

By the fourth time by the fifth enema you will some people become addicted. They enjoy this process so much. I can see for myself that even though I am an open minded person the first enema for me was pretty challenging but the second the third act like anything in life it gets easier and easier and easier. By the fourth or fifth time I was doing my enema I was literally hooked because of the feeling because of how easy it was and all my fears just disappeared into thin air. I was literally asking you know my mentor at the time if I could do it every day because this was something that was just magic. It just becomes second nature like brushing your teeth. So when people ask me and they say you know, can we do this process every week?" Can we do it on a consistent basis? Then I usually answer No and I will tell you why. Later on.

Enema Demonstration

This is an enema kit which contains two liters of liquid. We add and connect a hose on one and there is the connector to which the hose is connected like this. Okay. On the other side we take the small white tube and screw it on here like this here there is a faucet which is now closed and without looking at the faucet I can feel it and know that I have now opened it. Now it's 100 percent open and like this it's closed. Why am I showing you this? Because when we do an enema we don't really see the faucet with our eyes. We need to feed it. Soon you'll understand why okay. I suggest you practice opening and closing the faucet without looking in just by feeling it. Now I know it's open one hundred percent. And like this I know it's a little bit closed.

It's very important that the faucet is 100 percent open like this during the enema. After we have filled up the kit we go to the sink and lift up the kit with a tube mouth facing downwards towards the sink and we open the faucet slowly so the water pushes out all the air that's trapped in the hose at first. The water flow will filter until it begins to stabilize and flow freely. And then I know there is no air in the system. I closed the faucet and now I'm ready to do the enema. Okay so now that we filled up the kit with water I let the air out the hose will go and hang our kit in the highest place possible. You can also take a hanger and hook it onto the kit and then hang it from a door around this height and then the hose will nearly reach the floor.

Then what we need to do is lie down just like this. Okay as close as possible to the wall and then simply lift our legs up like so and take the to mouth and slowly insert into the—. We then open the faucet and the water will begin to flow into our body. The back with the fluids will slowly empty until the last pit stops. Just about here due to the law of gravity, we close a faucet and release the hose from our body. We then go into the cattle position and begin to shake our body a few times and then after a minute or two slowly bring our legs down and move into the next position. We now lie on our side, relax and get used to the feeling of the fluids inside slowly massage the stomach with the intention of taking the fluids into the center of the intestines.

After a minute or two of the massage we move into the six point position like so and shake our body like a dog does when they want to remove the excess water from their body we can then make waves with our stomach muscles before moving onto the next position. Now we lie on our right side and massage our stomachs here too. And after a minute or two it's recommended to move into the candle position again. Shake the body a few times and then slowly come down to the floor once again and move into the next position like previously and repeat the cycle as many times as you can. After we've done the cycle at least once we will head straight to the toilet and sit with our backs straight.

Not like we usually do of course and this is so that the fluids kind of flush out of our system as efficiently as possible. Also the flow of fluids that will come out will be strong and so will be the odor. There is a chance of nausea and a feeling of discomfort so Do not worry. There also may be some dizziness after the first wave of fluids does not just get up. You can even look into the toilet if you like just to see what came out. You may see a kind of white mucus, some small stones, even digestive food turned your body slightly to each side. And this allows more fluids to be released. Massage your stomach clockwise so that both fluids and gas that are left inside will all come out. What I would like to say is that the entire process for the hanging of the kit until the shower is around 30 minutes after all the fluids have left the system.

There is no chance that after an hour or so you'll have diarrhea or something like that. The enema. I suggest you do at night because usually after the enema the body becomes tired and wants to rest. Now if you feel exhausted after the enema I strongly suggest you do Another enema immediately afterwards because this is probably due to excess toxins which have not left our body and have entered our bloodstream and caused damage. Coffee enemas should only be done in the morning because if you do the coffee enema at night you will most likely not be able to sleep properly.

Apple Bonus

And now after a few days of our regime of rice and our first enema the bonus is now to take a sour green apple and to great it and enjoy this delicious delicious taste that is new to our taste buds. Because we reset and sometimes after the first enema we feel a feeling of hunger. The sour apple is a great way to give our body the feeling and taste that it's looking for. We don't want to give our body too much of itt. We don't want to put too much pressure on the body after the enema. After a few days of the progress that we've made, the apple is a nice treat to give yourself and you will be surprised at how delicious it will taste even though you may prefer the green apples or tastier fruit salad. Green apples will be tastier than you've ever had before. Believe me.

After the enema

So for those of you who did your first enema How was it? How do you feel afterwards? Do you feel relieved? Do you feel energized? Did your partner give you compliments on how quiet you were during the night? No snoring. Do you feel that you have more clarity? Maybe you've shed some pounds and kilograms from your stomach. You know how you feel. How is your general feeling if you have any questions for us. Obviously we are here. You can send it to us and we will reply within 24 hours. It's important for you to understand that thousands of people are going through the same process as you. You are not alone. So any feelings you have are obviously yours.

They are unique but they are common with everyone else. So do not be afraid to send us your questions. We will reply as soon as you send them to us. One also important point is that after the enema you may not feel a need to go to the toilet for maybe even a couple of days. That is completely natural. It's mainly because most of the toxins have been washed out of the body and the food that you are now consuming after the enema your body is using for energy. And so it's very precise. So there's very little waste being dumped outside which is. So it's important you understand this is not constipation. There's no need to worry if you do feel the need to consult with us and send us a question feel free to do so. We are here.

Some words of encouragement

OK. Great job. We have got through the hardest part of the process. We've gone through three days of literally surviving, you know, difficult situations mentally physically. I know how hard it is for you. Believe me I've been through this process many times before. And the hardest part is literally behind you okay. If you've got through this part the rest of the process will be a lot easier for you and I'm sure that it's already started to show you signs of improvement in various parts of your life maybe even in other areas of your life maybe in your personal life at work perhaps. And I know from my experience that it affects all areas of your life because it literally forces you to change your habits that have been embedded in you since you were a baby.

You know your eating habits or your emotional connections to your food and to sleep. And my first process you know I was literally cured of snoring for life. And this was after I did various surgeries on my nose and I tried various medications. The enema for me cured this. So I'm sure and I'm positive this is affecting you positively in other areas of your life. If you see small changes if no changes or appear don't worry they will begin to show up in the next few days because as I said you've got through the hardest part and I'm very proud of you to get that you've got this far. So let's move on.

Day 4

On the fourth day of the process we will add to the boring rice steamed carrot. What we will do is we will peel the carrot and chop it up into small pieces or we can grate it. And we want it to steam the carrot so that it's a nice texture and we can add that to the rice. It will add a lot of flavor. It will be the tastiest carrots you've ever had in your life. I promise you and this delicious meal is your first of many that will continue to come over the next few days. Obviously there is no limit to how much rice and carrot you can eat as much as you like. Every time you are hungry just whip up a meal and you're ready to go. In order to steam the carrot you couldn't use a cold on the inside of a saucepan. Make sure that the water does not touch the carrot when you're cooking it and you cook it for about 20 minutes until the texture is just right. Strain the water and you have your meal ready to go.

Days 5-7

On the fifth day of the process we add pumpkin to the carrot and the steamed cooked rice and this is basically to give us the sweet taste of the vegetables which we have not enjoyed for the first few days and also the the job of the orange vegetables is to basically clean the spleen which when it's out of balance allows our body to to host the parasites which are which are present in our digestive system and also the orange vegetables what they do is they clear out the veal they they basically helped to detox the liver and to detox our body as well. On the sixth day we will add the root of parsley and parsley to the carrot and to the pumpkin steamed and the cooked rice. And slowly slowly we are adding more and more vegetables and fruit as we progress.

The root of parsley just like the root of celery which will be added on the seventh day will give us that natural taste of salt which is in nature and it will also help to cleanse out our gallbladder, our urinary tract and our liver. On the seventh day we add to our diet the celery the root of the celery and the celery leaves to the other vegetables that we've had and at the end of the day after we've gone to the toilet or done a small mini enema to release the toxins we do our next enema with the camomile and the lemon foam today will start to consume the unique supplements which will help us with the process. The supplements will serve us three main purposes. The first is to restore balance to our body as a result of the end of the termination of all the parasites.

The second reason is to release the the desires the cravings for the sugars for the carbs and the third reason is to keep maintain our body weight which we have worked so hard on for the last seven days and we will continue to over the process of this detox in order to safely ensure that we have rid of all of the parasites in our body. We will take the supplements for a minimum of two months up to six months and this will as I say ensure that we are rid of all of the parasites in our system and that they will not return ever again. Instructions regarding the supplements how to take them when to take them you will receive in a separate sheet which is provided in this Book you can download and it's provided the link has provided for your convenience.

Days 8-11

On the eighth day of the process we will add a protein and the most recommended protein is egg. Now we suggest that you start with two eggs. Although some people will have a desire for law, the reason that we say start with two is because over the years some people have discovered that they have some kind of intolerance for certain foods after the detox process. And this is due to the reset of the system and because the body becomes now a clean canvas. It basically reacts to new foods as we introduce them and we straightaway we can identify which are good for us and which are not so weak. We recommend starting with two eggs.

The whole egg with the yolk as well and obviously because our body is kind of sensitive right now the best forms of eggs will be an omelet or poached egg soft egg not hard boiled because the system is going to have a difficult time in processing the hard boiled egg and this is obviously in addition to the rice and the steamed vegetables that we've already been eating so far for the vegans amongst us instead of the egg we can substitute it with tofu or with lentils or with sprouted mash. And if we are eating eggs then I do recommend that you use a very high quality saucepan, do not fry in butter, use some kind of oil like coconut oil or any other high quality oil on the ninth day. The process we can say goodbye to our beloved rice and we can now introduce quinoa with a quinoa.

We can begin to cook our vegetables together and then we can also slowly introduce some spices, maybe some cooking in some black pepper, some Cuban just a small amount and see how we react. Remember that the quinoa serves as a protein so it's a great source of nutrients during this process and it's also very tasty as well after we've been eating the rice for a whole week. On the 11th day of the process we can now have an orange soup and by orange I mean pumpkin sweet potatoes carrots and we can also add in the vegetables that we've been eating until now. The parsley and the celery and if you like you can throw in the rice or the Kino into the soup as well.

And that also added some some some interests and texture and make sure that you stay away from orange peppers OK no orange peppers we can add also now as a daily source of protein any kind of fish and with some lemon and some green herbs also we need to remember that we do not add salt at this point because the salt will will stop our process of losing weight. So please keep that in mind.

Days 12-14

On the 12th day of the process we can introduce a salad which will be composed from all the various green leaves arugula lettuce parsley can have the spinach and also add to it. Olive oil lemon juice. Also we can have introduced two types of proteins so any sources of protein or tofu or mash chicken nuts meat all these kinds of proteins. Obviously we will provide you with a list of proteins that will be good for you. And these you can introduce as I say slowly so that you give yourself a chance to recognize whether they are good for you. Whether they are not also will provide for you a specialized blood type sheet which will show you all the foods that you should or shouldn't be eating according to your blood type.

This is based on years and years of research and this will be a precious form of information for you and it's helped thousands of people before and I'm sure it will help you too. On the 30th day of the process we can add to our diet or replace any kind of grains or lagoons that you can basically find anything like oatmeal millet Amaranth. These are great sources of nutrients but remember to stay away from gluten so foods like Bruegel and semolina even spelt flour which is considered a very healthy form of flour. It actually still is gluten and we want to stay away from that so stick with this plan and you'll be good on the 13th day. We can add legumes and grains so oatmeal or anything like millet and we can have that frugal but remember to stay away from remember to stay away from the from the from the flour and from the wheat so we stick staying away from things like semolina you know even spelt flour. It contains gluten.

We're staying away from that for now by the 14th day we're already in this kind of strict you know precise regime. And basically it can get a bit boring and dull. So we can alternate the way that we're cooking our food and we can start to cook in the oven. We can perhaps make a stew combined, change the mix and and change the combinations of the foods that we're eating and we can also introduce some other kinds of food like wild rice colored quinoa. And this will add a bit of variation to our diet.

Coffee enema and passive weight loss

We finished 14 days of the process. Amazing job. Now we move on to the next enema which will be coffee enema. Yes. Yes. People, it's going to be a coffee enema. The sixth and the seventh enema will be with coffee. And let me explain to you how it is done. We will take the black coffee, preferably Turkish coffee if you can get a hold of it. We take five teaspoons of the black coffee and we boil two liters of water and we let the coffee sit in the water for a number of hours. Once the coffee has then sunk to the bottom we will drain the liquid and what will remain is just the pure coffee without the bits of the black the black coffee.

Basically we suggest from our experience that

you do the coffee enema in the morning and this is due to the content of the caffeine because we do want to sleep at night which is why we do not do the enema in the evening. The benefits of the coffee enema are highly highly effective. So stick with us and you will see why the coffee enema is such a great part of this process. So it's been two weeks since the beginning of the process and it is time to take another picture of ourselves and of our tongue and compare to how it was from the beginning of the process. Now the main purpose of this whole process as by its name is for a detox that is a primary purpose that we are during this process. Although some of you may have entered this process as a source of losing weight, that is actually a byproduct too.

And this is where the term passive loss of weight comes in because as I said this is a byproduct of the detox process and as we continue with this whole routine we will see that as we are detoxing our body as a natural side effect it basically will lose weight. And this is why we call it passive because we are not doing sport. You know we're not taking anything that is chemical to help to shed those pounds kilograms from our body. We are basically just stopping the toxins from coming and releasing them from our body and out. We're letting our system do the job by itself naturally and this is why we call it passive. We have one week left to go and by now I am positive that you are already seeing the positive effects that it's had on your life on your system. And I'm sure that you've come this far. What's another week? You know it's just a few days left and the process once it's complete you'll be good to go you know and go on your own and continue this process by yourself.

Recipes?

Before we continue with the process I would like to make an important point here. The reason that we do not include recipes in this process is because everybody has their own taste. So what we do provide are basically sheets that have all the foods that are allowed according to blood type. Obviously the foods that are allowed are not allowed and neutral for the parasites for the parasite cleansing. We leave it up to you to basically make your own meals according to your own personal taste you know. And as I've said many times before, as soon as you have something that disagrees with your body you will know immediately. And this is something that is new from this body detox process that you've never experienced before.

Due to all the toxins in your body your body now is like clean sheets or anything new that will agitate your system. You will know immediately and you'll be able to cut it out from your life. Start off your morning with a rich breakfast in protein and vegetables because breakfast is the most important meal of the day. It's what gives you the juice and the energy for the day. And I also recommend that you make sure you have enough time to eat your breakfast. And you know even if you're not accustomed to having a big breakfast in the morning I strongly suggest that you find the time and this after you begin to see the results. I promise you that you will not want to give this up.

Stick to it

So as we've said previously you know at this stage we've already lost most of our old habits and we've started a new routine. Now this is not the time to grow back. We want to progress. And even though sometimes the urge is strong you may walk past a bakery you may see other people you know eating foods that you miss. But I promise you that if we continue it will be worth it in the long run because remember the time when you would just sit down with a cup of coffee you know and have a question or some kind of sandwich and while the taste was good it wasn't long lasting. But what was long lasting were the effects on your body.

And once we've developed these new habits our system has started to reset itself and it's benefiting from all these nutrients. And we want to stick with it. We want to move forward and we will see more results coming with time. In order to keep this good feeling and in order to maintain this whole process we just stick to the routine. We stick to the plan and we will consume these supplements for another two months at least so that we will receive the maximum effect desired.

Conclusion

Congratulations. We've reached day 21 of the detox process. This is time now for another coffee enema. And like we said before , the coffee enema we do in the morning time so that we do not interfere with our sleep in the evening. We've explained before how to do the coffee enema so you can follow those instructions and we're ready to go. So is this the end of the process? Well on one hand it is but on the other hand it's the beginning of a new life for you. You've received here an amazing tool box for life that you can use and that you should use after this whole detox has finished.

You know sometimes we have the tendency to go back to old habits but I strongly advise that you continue with this routine for as long as you possibly can because we want to maintain these new levels of energy you know the new skin that's radiating and I'm sure by now you're receiving new compliments on how you're looking and I'm not even talking about how you're feeling you know we'll focus sleeping better more energy levels your memory has maybe improved a little bit and you know after you've discovered which foods are good for you and which foods are not. And you've also seen that you can live off a third of the foods that you were before and have even higher energy levels. I'm sure you see the benefits of sticking with this diet and continuing in order to live an energetic and healthy lifestyle.

Important message over the next three months. We want to stick to our optimal precise diet. OK. And as I said before we're providing you with the lists of the parasite foods and the blood type foods that are beneficial that are detrimental. And the foods that are neutral now there is one point that is very important that I need to clarify. If you look according to the sheet of the parasites and it is allowed. But on the sheet of the blood type it is not allowed. Then we do not eat it. And the obviously vice versa if on the blood sheet it is allowed. But on the parasite sheet it is not allowed.

We also do not eat it. I strongly suggest over the first two months that we stick to neutral foods and we will see how our body reacts and then only after the third month we start to introduce new foods that we can try and test on ourselves and see how it reacts. As I've said numerous times this is a new life for you and I know that for some of you it is. Well it's not for some of you is actually one of us. You know where we're human beings, we have our lives, we have all kinds of events that we attend. And sometimes it can be challenging. You know we go to an event and there's a birthday party and there's cakes and there's alcohol and you know go to a coffee shop and there's bread and there's questions and bakeries and everywhere we have everywhere we go there are basically you know we have temptations.

And if a desire is to have one of these foods you know and to live a little bit then obviously be my guest. And just know that you have this toolset that will help you in order to reset your system to how it is now when it goes out of balance. So if you see it all that's fine. Just make sure that you get back into your center into your balance that your body has come now accustomed to. No. And this is basically a tool box being given.

It's easy you know and it's up to you. So all I can say to you now is good luck on your journey. Thank you for joining us. And it was an incredible process. And I'm sure that this will change your life for the better. Good luck. See you soon.

Don't miss out!

Visit the website below and you can sign up to receive emails whenever Gaurav Sanjiv Kalangan publishes a new book. There's no charge and no obligation.

https://books2read.com/r/B-A-EPFBB-JMWZC

Also by Gaurav Sanjiv Kalangan

Learn Options Strategies Options Basics & Greeks For Stock Trading By Technical Analysis

Bitcoin, Altcoins & ICOs Learn the Basics of Digital Coins from Zero

Time Management This Is How I Work 300 Percent Faster

How To Build And Implement A Winning Pricing Strategy

Networking For Introverts: Gracefully Exiting A Conversation

Accounting 101: Learn Cost Accounting From A To Z

Growth Marketing: Strategy & Execution Bootcamp For Startups

Develop The Mental Strength Of A Warrior For Success In Life

Time Management Mastery: Productivity & Goals

Complete Fitness Trainer Certification: Beginner To Advanced